JUVENILE RHEUMATOID ARTHRITIS

Edited by
John J. Miller, III

PSG Publishing Company, Inc.
Littleton, Massachusetts

Library of Congress Cataloging in Publication Data
Main entry under title:

Juvenile rheumatoid arthritis.

    Includes index.
    1. Rheumatoid arthritis in children. I. Miller,
John Johnston, 1934-   [DNLM: 1. Arthritis,
Juvenile rheumatoid. WE346 J97]
RJ482.A77J88   618.9′27′2   78-55290
ISBN 0-88416-189-7

Printed in the United States of America

International Standard Book Number: 0-88416-189-7

Library of Congress Catalog Card Number: 78-55290

CONTRIBUTORS

Bram H. Bernstein, M.D.
Associate Clinical Professor of
  Pediatrics
University of Southern California
Division of Rheumatology
Children's Hospital of Los Angeles
Los Angeles, California

Leo T. Chylack, Jr., M.D.
Assistant Professor of
  Ophthalmology
Harvard Medical School
Howe Laboratory of
  Ophthalmology
Massachusetts Eye and Ear
  Infirmary
Boston, Massachusetts

William H. Donovan, M.D.
Assistant Professor
Department of Rehabilitation
  Medicine
University of Washington
Seattle, Washington

David K. Dueker, M.D.
Instructor in Ophthalmology
Harvard Medical School
Massachusetts Eye and Ear
  Infirmary
Boston, Massachusetts

Linda J. Gorin, M.D.
Lecturer in Pediatrics
University of California at Davis
Davis, California

J. Roger Hollister, M.D.
Assistant Professor of Pediatrics
University of Colorado
National Jewish Hospital and
  Research Center
Denver, Colorado

Mark Johnson, Ph.D.
Clinical Psychologist
Pediatric Service
Rancho Los Amigos Hospital
Downey, California

Deborah W. Kredich, M.D.
Assistant Professor of Pediatrics
Duke University School of Medicine
Durham, North Carolina

Carol B. Lindsley, M.D.
Assistant Professor of Pediatrics
The University of Kansas College of
  Health Sciences
Kansas City, Kansas

**Andrew J. McMichael, M.B., Ph.D.,
M.R.C.P.**
Wellcome Senior Research Fellow
Nuffield Department of Clinical
  Medicine
The Radcliff Infirmary
Oxford University
Oxford, United Kingdom

John J. Miller, III, M.D., Ph.D.
Associate Professor of Clinical
  Pediatrics
The Children's Hospital at Stanford
Stanford University School of
  Medicine
Stanford, California

Lauren M. Pachman, M.D.
Professor of Pediatrics
The Children's Memorial Hospital
Northwestern University
Chicago, Illinois

Ross E. Petty, M.D.
Associate Professor of Pediatrics
Children's Center
The University of Manitoba
Winnipeg, Manitoba, Canada

Donovan J. Pihlaja, Ph.D.
Instructor in Ophthalmic Research
Harvard Medical School
Boston, Massachusetts

Lawrence A. Rinsky, M.D.
Assistant Professor of Orthopaedics
The Children's Hospital at Stanford
Stanford University School of
  Medicine
Stanford, California

Bernhard H. Singsen, M.D.
Assistant Clinical Professor of
  Pediatrics

University of Southern California
Division of Rheumatology
Children's Hospital of Los Angeles
Los Angeles, California

David A. Stempel, M.D.
Assistant Professor of Pediatrics
University of North Carolina
Chapel Hill, North Carolina

Donald M. Thompson, M.D.
Senior Fellow
Division of Rheumatology
Children's Hospital of Los Angeles
Los Angeles, California

CONTENTS

PREFACE

I hesitated when I was first asked to start this book. The subject of "juvenile rheumatoid arthritis" has been long neglected in comparison to forms of arthritis in adults, but in the last several years there has been a heartening increase in the numbers of journal articles, conferences, and monographs on the subject. Although formal training programs are few and far between, and although their numbers are small, pediatric rheumatologists have recently gained places of respect in the councils of the American Rheumatism Association and at The International Congresses of Rheumatology.

To create a book which would add to, rather than just duplicate, existing literature, I have tried two strategies. First, I have picked younger or emerging contributors with the hope that new points of view would be expressed; "professors" and the "establishment" (if such exists) were excluded. Secondly, all the authors were asked to emphasize the current state of the science of their subject. Unhappily this is often limited. A constant theme throughout the book is the narrow range of our knowledge in regard to arthritis in children or in growing animals, in contrast to adult forms of arthritis.

Whether or not new perspectives have been presented will have to be a judgment of the reader. Obviously the biases of the authors reflect the sources of their training and inspiration. I am indebted for my scientific attitudes to J. Lowell Orbison and John Vaughan at The University of Rochester and, later, at The Scripps Institute in La Jolla and to Gustav J.V. Nossal in Melbourne. My clinical training was with Gordon Williams and Niels Brandstrup who developed the program in pediatric rheumatology at Stanford. Amongst the other authors, Linda Gorin, Carol Lindsley, Roger Hollister and William Donovan have had part of their training at Seattle under Jane Schaller, Ralph Wedgwood, and Mart Mannik. Bram Bernstein, Bern Singsen and Donald Thompson have worked extensively in Virgil Hanson's program in Los Angeles. Ross Petty was long associated with Donita Sullivan and James Cassidy at Michigan. Andrew McMichael and David Stempel were working in Hugh McDevitt's laboratory at Stanford when asked to write their chapter. The other contributors appear, at least to me, to have developed their interests and particular prejudices quite independently.

A major problem has been to decide about the title of the book and the categorization of the clinical descriptions. "Juvenile rheumatoid arthritis" (JRA), is the currently favored term for this subject in the

United States, while "juvenile chronic polyarthropathy" (JCP) is preferred in England and appears to be making gains in Europe and in the United States. I chose the former because, although in danger of going out of style, it still is universally recognized. The use of the John Calabro- and Jane Schaller-inspired categories of "systemic," "polyarticular," and "pauciarticular," instead of the English system (see Chapter 1) is due to the biases induced by my more frequent contact with United States workers. However, my intuitive reaction is to reject categorization by clinical manifestations. More than one pathogenic mechanism is almost certainly responsible for the collected syndromes called JRA or JCP. I strongly suspect that when these mechanisms are defined we will find overlapping clinical features due to different basic events, and that little of the nomenclature used in this book will persist.

Finally, I want to state that I have tried to interfere as little as possible with the contributions of each author. This has led to the disadvantage of duplication of material among chapters, but also to the advantage that each chapter can stand alone as a complete review of its subject.

John J. Miller III
December, 1977

SECTION I

Basic Mechanisms: Current Scientific Knowledge

1 History, Folklore, Current Controversy

Deborah W. Kredich and
John J. Miller III

THE ANTIQUITY OF ARTHRITIS

Joint diseases have afflicted man since ancient times.[1,2] Egyptian mummies show convincing evidence of ankylosing spondylitis, osteoarthritis, and gout. During the time of Hippocrates these diseases were considered together under the general term "rheumatismas," meaning inflammation of joints.[1] It was thought that circulating evil humors formed into a mucus catarrh, settling into the joints and producing inflammation. Through the ages, "rheumatism" afflicted many famous people. It is said that Pope Pius II was unable to go on the last crusade against the Turks because of joint disease; Christopher Columbus was apparently very crippled; and Mary Queen of Scots was carried in a chair because of her severe joint disease. Other famous persons afflicted by one joint disorder or another included James Madison and Pierre Renoir. However, distinctions between gout, rheumatoid arthritis, and osteoarthritis were not made until relatively recently.

Among Syndenham's voluminous writings during the last half of the seventeenth century is a description of the typical hyperextension deformities of the proximal interphalangeal joints associated with adult-onset rheumatoid arthritis.[2] This appears to be ample evidence for the existence of rheumatoid arthritis distinct from other arthritides at that time. However, Short expresses the opinion that the peripheral joint deformities found in Egyptian mummies and other ancient human remains are simply representative of the peripheral arthopathy seen in ankylosing spondylitis.[2] Whether or not rheumatoid arthritis existed in ancient times or whether tophaceous gout and severe early-onset osteoarthritis were the main offenders in terms of joint disease in the ancients, significant joint disease has obviously been an important aspect of man's history.

FOLKLORE

There are numerous recurring themes in man's assessment of the etiology and treatment of arthritis. One of the foremost is nutrition. Hippocrates treated gout with a diet avoiding certain high protein foods.[3] Today one of the popular prevailing notions is that rheumatoid arthritis is in large part due to allergy or other forms of intolerance to food. There are numerous physicians and others who propose treatment of rheumatoid arthritis and juvenile rheumatoid arthritis (JRA) with various elimination diets. Many patients with JRA also have allergies and it is certainly possible that in a few patients allergies contribute to the general ill health of the patient. Unfortunately, some of the proponents of diets also preach elimination of aspirin and other beneficial treatment. Additions to the diet have been advocated for years and a wide variety of vitamin supplements is recommended in many currently popular regimens. Cod liver oil to lubricate stiff joints, was frequently given with orange juice but one wonders whether such therapy gained credence from results in patients suffering from the bone pain of scurvy or rickets. A best-selling book by D.C. Jarvis[4] advocated daily use of apple cider vinegar and honey. Part of the philosophy behind this therapy was that the acidity of the vinegar would dissolve calcium around stiff joints and that the honey would help to hold calcium in solution. Jarvis also recommended, as do many current nutritionists, increasing the use of natural foods and decreasing intake of animal protein.[4]

Another recurring theme for therapy of arthritis has been to remove the "focus of infection" theoretically responsible for the disease. In ancient times extractions of teeth were commonly performed. More recently tonsillectomies, adenoidectomies, cholecystectomies, and sinus irrigations have been done in an attempt to cure arthritis. Purges have been popular in this regard through the ages.[1]

It has long been recognized that fever or acute stress have preceded remissions of rheumatoid arthritis. Milk protein injections have been used in an attempt to promote fever, and even epinephrine has been tried.[1] Bee keepers have been noted to be free of rheumatoid arthritis since early Roman times and from this grew the theories promoting bee venom therapy.[5] Indeed, bee venom injections have proven effective in experimental models of arthritis, but not in adrenalectomized animals. The effect is probably mediated by adrenal steroids.

In ancient Rome the physician Scribonius recommended that his patients frequent a beach where there were numerous torpedo fish. The arthritic patient would place his feet on the torpedo fish and experience electric shock. In the eighteenth century, Michael Faraday designed the Faradic coil to stimulate underused muscles around stiff joints. Beneficial results occurring in some of his patients led to the rapid growth of loosely related enterprises involving magnetic belts, magnetic rings, and charms. More recently there was a suggestion that radiation might have similar positive effects and "uranitoriums" abounded in the 1950s. People paid great sums of money in order to sit in mine shafts where "beneficial radiation" was supposed to reach them.[1]

The relaxing and soothing effects of heat and massage in patients with stiff or painful joints and muscles have also been appreciated since ancient times. Spas, taking advantage of natural hot springs, pleasant surroundings, etc., have prospered since the early Romans.

Obviously, some of these treatments are indeed helpful. The time-honored modalities of heat and controlled exercises still form the cornerstones of our approach to the treatment of the child with JRA. Numerous other therapies certainly do no harm: the wearing of a copper bracelet, the use of vitamin supplements in moderation, the use of vinegar and honey as a tonic, or acupuncture. Until the "cure" is found it is important that the physician caring for the child afflicted with the disease be tolerant of the nonmedical forms of therapy that the families and friends of such patients will continue to try. It is not unreasonable for parents to consider copper bracelets as similar to gold injections or the swallowing of zinc.[6] At the same time dangerous fads and emotional overinvestment in useless or expensive therapies must be warned against.

PEDIATRIC RHEUMATOLOGY

The origins of pediatric rheumatology are generally attributed to Sir George Frederick Still, the first professor of pediatrics in the history of Great Britain,[7,8] in a paper which was presented and discussed in 1896 but not published until 1897.[9,10] However, Short discusses a thesis by a French medical student, Landre-Beauvais, written in 1800, which described deforming arthritis in young females with a prolonged disease course and impaired motion of the joints.[2] Bywaters was able to find a number of reports of arthritis in children from France, Brazil, and New York in the period between 1864 and 1869. However, Still did present the first definitive paper of JRA in which he detailed descriptions of 19 cases which he had personally observed.[8-11] Among these can be found examples of the various subtypes of JRA that we recognize today. Six of the patients had arthritis that appeared very like that in rheumatoid adults with "bony grating," generalized enlargement of the joints, and progressive deformities. They did not have systemic aspects of disease such as splenomegaly, pericarditis, or enlarged lymph nodes and there were no deaths in the group. Twelve others had progressive and severe joint deformities with associated systemic symptoms including enlargement of lymph nodes and spleen, early onset of disease, severe pericarditis, and prominent fever. He also described growth problems and made a special point that the patients he observed had normal mentality. He observed that intercurrent infections often resulted in improvement of the joint disease. It was Still's feeling that rheumatoid arthritis in children represented an infectious process. In a major textbook of pediatrics he made no mention of this disease.

Much important and detailed chronicling of arthritis in children has been done by twentieth century rheumatologists in England. Of major importance for the world was the founding of the Rheumatism Research Unit in the Canadian Red Cross Memorial Hospital at Taplow, England in 1947. The group of physicians and scientists who have worked in this unit has contributed more to our understanding of JRA than has any other single source. Most prominent, at least to pediatric rheumatologists, among those who have worked at Taplow are E.G.L. Bywaters (who has written a witty and informative chronicle of the early days of pediatric rheumatology[7]), Barbara Ansell, and John Holborow. Unfortunately for the rest of us the unit has recently been disbanded, although most of its members are active.

An increased interest in chronic childhood arthritis also appeared in Europe following World War II. Scandinavia produced important clinical studies by Edstrom and Sury.[12,13] Probably the most comprehensively studied large series of patients presented in a single report is that by Anna-Lisa Laaksonen from Turku, Finland.[14] More recently, Norway has become a center of active immunological research in JRA by several workers including Munthe, Hoyerral, Froland, and Natvig (see Chapter 4).

In the United States interest in JRA also grew during the 1940s.

This was probably due in part to the declining incidence of acute rheumatic fever. "Convalescent" hospitals for children such as La Rabida in Chicago, Sea Shore House in Atlantic City, and those associated with the Children's Hospital of Los Angeles and Stanford University, began to pay more attention to patients with chronic arthritis as fewer patients with rheumatic fever were admitted. In addition, immunologists became interested in the collagen diseases, and internist-rheumatologists became interested in children. Early papers in the United States included those of Coss and Boots and of Lockie and Norcross.[15,16] Comprehensive monographs appeared in 1962 and 1970.[17,18]

Worldwide interest has finally reached a level which has resulted in productive international meetings concerned solely or predominantly with the subject of children's arthritis.[19-21] American Rheumatism Association meetings now devote at least one half-day to pediatric subjects.

CONTROVERSIES

Increased attention has produced new knowledge which, however, has remained well behind that of the adult arthritides. It has also produced some healthy controversy. Since we are still in a stage of developing clinical description and classification, most of the current arguments concern criteria and nomenclature. A committee of the American Rheumatism Association has developed tentative criteria for diagnosis of JRA which follow the American system of classification, but its value is questioned in England, and the Taplow group has adopted an entirely different nomenclature.[22]

The American scheme was first presented forcefully by John Calabro[23] but has been most refined and popularized by Jane Schaller[24] and Ralph Wedgwood and has received the approval of the American Rheumatism Association. It is the system used in this book, based on the *clinical* mode of onset during the first six months. *Systemic* JRA is that form of disease usually called Still's disease in the United States. The criteria require daily intermittent fever to 103°F., and rash, adenopathy, splenomegaly, anemia, and leukocytosis are common. *Polyarticular* JRA is that with five or more joints involved, but with less severe fever. *Pauciarticular* JRA is that involving four or fewer joints. This classification has some prognostic usefulness and is a convenient way of describing patients. However, it lacks scientific or pathologic rationale. Attempts are just starting to define subgroups by the presence of abnormal antibodies or distinctive leukocyte antigens.[25] However, currently used laboratory parameters have, at best, good but never absolute correlations with the clinical state.

Bywaters, Ansell, and their group have proposed, and use, another system.[26-28] Their scheme is also based on clinical appearances, but those which are seen late in the disease. They use the generic name "juvenile chronic polyarthritis" (JCP). *Juvenile rheumatoid arthritis* is applied only to those children who have a positive test for rheumatoid factor. *Ankylosing spondylitis* is included in this group since its onset may be indistinguishable. The remaining two types are *JCP 1) with, or 2) without, sacroiliitis.* The former has the presumed potential to progress to ankylosing spondylitis and shares a high incidence of HLA-B27 positivity. Within this scheme, the terms "systemic" or "pauciarticular" are used to describe a patient's disease at a given point in time. This classification puts more stress on the worst outcomes and it is intuitively difficult to accept such terminology for those children with the more benign and remittent courses. It does use laboratory and radiography data to define the subgroups and thus may have better correlation with still unknown pathogenic mechanisms. Other problems which remain controversial will be covered in subsequent chapters.

Our general lack of good scientific information is an ongoing theme throughout the book. The role of infection, direct or indirect, is still argued; T cells, B cells, or both may be causing synovitis; an array of inflammatory biologic materials is being identified but the relative importance of each group of substances within joints is totally unknown.

Clearly we are just at the beginning of the history of pediatric rheumatology.

REFERENCES

1. Corrigan, A.B. *Living with Arthritis.* Edited by Alan Tengove. Sydney: Murray, 1969.
2. Short, C.L. The antiquity of rheumatoid arthritis. *Arthritis Rheum.* 17:193–205, 1974.
3. Hernden, B. Diet in the treatment of rheumatoid disease. *Am J Clin Nutr.* 18:68–74, 1966.
4. Jarvis, D.C. *Arthritis and Folk Medicine.* New York: Holt, Reinhart, and Winston, 1960.
5. Broadman, J. *Bee Venom: The Natural Curative for Arthritis and Rheumatism.* New York: G.P. Putnam Sons, 1962.
6. Simkin, P.A. Oral zinc sulphate in rheumatoid arthritis. *Lancet* 2:539–42, 1976.
7. Bywaters, E.G.L. The history of pediatric rheumatology. *Arthritis Rheum.* 20 (suppl):145–52, 1977.
8. Birch, C.A. Still's Disease: George Frederick Still. *The Practitioner.* 210:307–8, 1973.

9. Still, G.F. A form of chronic joint disease in children. *Br Med J.* 2:1446–7, 1896.

10. Still, G.F. On a form of chronic joint disease in children. *Med Chir Trans.* 80:47–60, 1897.

11. Still, G.F. *Common Disorders and Diseases of Childhood.* London: Oxford University Press, First Edition, 1909 through Fifth Edition, 1927.

12. Edstrom, G. Rheumatoid arthritis in children; clinical study. *Acta Paediatr.* 34:334–56, 1947.

13. Sury, B. Rheumatoid arthritis in children. A clinical study. *Thesis.* Copenhagen: Munksgaar, 1952.

14. Laaksonen, A.-L. A prognostic study of juvenile rheumatoid arthritis. *Acta Paediatr Scand.* 166 (suppl):1–163, 1966.

15. Coss, J., and Boots, J.H. Juvenile rheumatoid arthritis. *J Pediatr.* 29:143–56, 1946.

16. Lockie, L.M., and Norcross, B.M. Juvenile rheumatoid arthritis. *Pediatrics.* 2:694–8, 1948.

17. Grokoest, A.W., Synder, A.I., and Schlaeger, R. *Juvenile Rheumatoid Arthritis.* Boston: Little, Brown, 1961.

18. Brewer, E.J., Jr. *Juvenile Rheumatoid Arthritis.* Philadelphia: W.B. Saunders Co., 1970.

19. Seminar on the Role of the Orthopaedist in the Management of Juvenile Rheumatoid Arthritis. Glen Cove, New York, April, 1972.

20. First American Rheumatism Association Conference on the Rheumatic Diseases of Childhood. Park City, Utah, March, 1976.

21. EULAR/W.H.O. Workshop on the care of rheumatic children. Oslo, Norway, Jan. 1977.

22. Brewer, E.J., Jr., Bass, J., Baum, J. et al. Current Proposed Revision of JRA Criteria. *Arthritis Rheum.* 20 (suppl):195–9, 1977.

23. Calabro, J.J., and Marchesano, J.M. The early natural history of juvenile rheumatoid arthritis. *Med Clin North Am.* 52:567–91, 1968.

24. Schaller, J.G., and Wedgwood, R.J. Juvenile rheumatoid arthritis: a review. *Pediatrics.* 50:940–53, 1972.

25. Schaller, J.G. The diversity of JRA. *Arthritis Rheum.* 20 (suppl):S52–S61, 1977.

26. Edmonds, J., Morris, R.I., Metzger, A.L. et al. Follow-up study of juvenile chronic polyarthritis with particular reference to histocompatibility antigen W27. *Ann Rheum Dis.* 33:289–92, 1974.

27. Ansell, B.M. Juvenile chronic polyarthritis. Series 3. *Arthritis Rheum.* 20 (suppl):176–8, 1977.

28. Bywaters, E.G.L., Ansell, B.M., and Wood, P.H.N. Nomenclature and classification of juvenile chronic polyarthritis, abstracted. *Scand J Rheumatol.* 4 (suppl 8):34–02, 1975.

2 Epidemiology of Juvenile Rheumatoid Arthritis

Ross E. Petty

Epidemiology was first systematically applied to the study of rheumatic diseases in Great Britain by Glover.[1] In this and later surveys, adult populations with rheumatic diseases were studied, however, individuals below the age of 15 years were excluded. As a result there are few data relating to the epidemiology of the rheumatic diseases in childhood. In addition, derivation of valid epidemiologic data from evaluation of published studies of arthritis in childhood is made difficult by the absence of uniform diagnostic criteria.

DIAGNOSTIC CRITERIA AND CLASSIFICATIONS

The term juvenile rheumatoid arthritis (JRA) has somewhat different meanings in different parts of the world. While there are valid reasons for favoring one or another classification, the differences (discussed in Chapter 1) must be understood in order to utilize data from various centers.[2,3] For the sake of clarity the following discussion of epidemiologic information will be presented in the context of the American Rheumatism Association proposed criteria, unless otherwise noted.

PREVALENCE AND INCIDENCE OF JRA

The prevalence of disease is an expression of the proportion of persons at risk (for example, within a certain age range), who have the disease. Bywaters estimated the prevalence of Still's disease (juvenile chronic polyarthritis) at 0.06% of an English school population.[4] The criteria used for diagnosis were onset before age 16, involvement of four or more joints for at least three months with either pain and swelling, pain and limitation of movement or limitation of movement and swelling. If fewer than four joints were involved, synovial membrane histology compatible with rheumatoid arthritis was required to make the diagnosis. In a questionnaire survey by Pless and Satterwhite, referred to by Baum,[5] a prevalence of 110 per 100,000 was determined. In a community survey in Tecumseh, Michigan,[6] two children under age 15 had definite or probable JRA, giving a prevalence very close to that determined by Bywaters. A second approach to determination of the prevalence of JRA is to compare relative frequency of JRA to RA in adults. Such ratios range from 1 in 100 to 5 or more in 100.[7,8] Using this type of calculation, Baum has suggested that there are at least 37,500 children in the United States with JRA.

The incidence of a disease refers to the number of new cases occurring in a specified time (usually one year) in the population at risk. In the study by Laaksonen an incidence of JRA based on hospitalized patients was estimated at 3.5 cases per 100,000 population at risk per year.[8] In a report by Sullivan, Cassidy and Petty, based on all children under 16 years of age with JRA, an incidence of 9.2 per 100,000 per year was calculated.[9]

Although these limited estimates are of variable validity and are somewhat conflicting it is probable that JRA has a minimal prevalence in the population below age 16 of approximately 66 per 100,000 and an annual incidence rate in the same age group of 9 per 100,000. At least 40,000 children in the United States have JRA and greater than 5000 develop the disease each year. These figures probably represent minimal estimates.

There are no data to enable determination of whether or not the incidence of JRA is increasing, decreasing, or remaining static. Although references to disease consistent with JRA are found in the literature of the nineteenth century there is increasing recognition of this disorder. Whether or not this is a result of an actual increase in disease incidence or of greater recognition and accuracy of diagnosis remains to be seen.

RACIAL AND GEOGRAPHIC ORIGIN

JRA has been recognized in all major racial groups and in temperate and tropical areas of the world. Some reports have suggested that rheumatoid arthritis in children and adults may be less common in African than in European populations, but that children may account for a greater proportion of the total affected population in Africa.[7] There have been no well-documented differences in the prevalence of JRA between American black and white populations; the observations by Hanson et al.[10] in a large population of children with JRA in the southwestern United States, that there were proportionately fewer black than white children with JRA, requires further study. Similarly, JRA may be relatively uncommon in North Americans of Chinese ancestry.[10,11] In contrast Hill has reported a higher incidence of JRA in the British Columbia Indian population (7.2/100,000/year) than in the Caucasian population (2.2/100,000/year), an observation which may reflect the high incidence of HLA-B27 and ankylosing spondylitis reported in the first group and the difficulty in differentiating early ankylosing spondylitis from pauciarticular JRA.[11,12]

SEX DISTRIBUTION AND AGE AT ONSET

In most large series of patients with JRA the ratio of girls to boys is approximately 2 or 3:1.[8,9,13,14] There are, however, several factors which can influence this overall ratio, two of the most important being age at onset and type of onset of disease. The age of onset of symptoms or signs consistent with a diagnosis of JRA has been examined in three large patient groups.[8,9,14] In all, a bimodal distribution of age at onset was observed. In two the early peak was between two and five years of age with a later peak at 10 to 15 years.[8,14] In the third study, in 300 children with JRA fulfilling the ARA proposed diagnostic criteria there was a peak age at onset between one and three years and a second broad peak between 7 and 11 years.[9] Comparison of age at onset of JRA to that of other rheumatic diseases of childhood is shown in Figure 1. The striking early peak distinguishes JRA from other rheumatic diseases.

Analysis of the second peak (between 7 and 11) reveals that it consists predominantly of boys (Figure 2), and in fact is similar to the

14

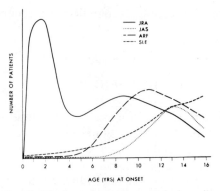

Figure 1. The relative distribution of age at onset in juvenile rheumatoid arthritis (JRA), juvenile ankylosing spondylitis (JAS), acute rheumatic fever (ARF), and systemic lupus erythematosus (SLE). Only JRA has a high incidence in the 1- to 3-year age group.

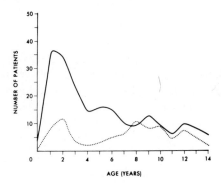

Figure 2. Distribution of age at onset of JRA in boys (. . . . . .) and girls (_____).

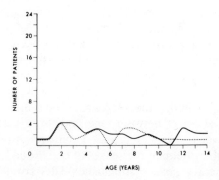

Figure 3. Distribution of age at onset of systemic JRA in boys (. . . . . .) and girls (_____).

age distribution for onset of juvenile ankylosing spondylitis.[15,16] An increased incidence of HLA-B27, a genetic marker strongly associated with ankylosing spondylitis, has been reported in the late onset group of patients indicating that this peak may include or consist of children with that condition.[17] When age at onset and sex ratios are examined for each onset subtype, differences are striking (Figures 3, 4, and 5). For children with JRA of systemic onset there is no peak age of onset. However, for those with pauciarticular or polyarticular onset there is the characteristic peak at one to three years of age and (for boys) at 7 to 11 years of age.

The sex composition of each of the modes of onset is also quite characteristic. In children with pauciarticular onset the ratio of girls to boys is 3.92:1. In those with polyarticular onset, girls outnumber boys

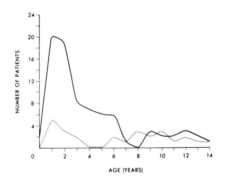

Figure 4. Distribution of age at onset of pauciarticular JRA in boys (. . . . . .) and girls (_____).

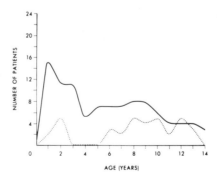

Figure 5. Distribution of age at onset of polyarticular JRA in boys (. . . . . .) and girls (_____).

2.84:1, but in those with systemic disease, the sex ratio is approximately equal (1.22:1).[9] The difference between sexes in incidence of iridocyclitis is also striking, the ratio of girls to boys ranging from 5:1 to 6.6:1 in three series.[18,19,20]

ENVIRONMENTAL INFLUENCES

No geographic aggregations of JRA have been noted to suggest any specific environmental influence. Lyme arthritis,[21] reported in a geographically restricted area of northeastern United States, is probably of infectious origin and unrelated to JRA. Other associations with infectious disease have been observed but the link with JRA is tenuous.[22-24]

FAMILY STUDIES

In general, JRA is not thought of as a familial disorder. In particular, its incidence in two or more first degree relatives is unusual. In a study of 277 relatives (siblings over 15 years of age, parents and grandparents) of 92 children with juvenile chronic polyarthritis, Ansell et al.[25] found a somewhat greater incidence of polyarthritis in female relatives and ankylosing spondylitis in the male relatives, than would have been expected in a normal population. It should be recalled, however, that the group of children included those with ankylosing spondylitis so the increased incidence of sacroiliac disease in male relatives is not unexpected. Only one of 92 children had an affected sibling who on follow-up had ankylosing spondylitis.

In the same study, 11 of 382 children with juvenile chronic polyarthritis were twins (2.6%), five monozygous and six dizygous. None of the dizygous twin pairs was concordant for JRA but two of the monozygous twin pairs were.[25] This number included some children who later were found to have ankylosing spondylitis so that the exact incidence of JRA in siblings or twins remains to be determined. There are no reports of the coincidence of JRA of different onset subtypes in the same sibship.

IMPLICATIONS OF EPIDEMIOLOGIC STUDIES

It might be expected that epidemiologic studies of a relatively uncommon chronic disease such as JRA would have led to knowledge of its cause or causes. To date, this has not been so. JRA remains a disease or diseases of unknown cause or causes, perhaps in part because epidemiologic studies have been limited. With common acceptance of diagnostic criteria, widespread use of serologic tests such as antinuclear antibody and rheumatoid factor, and exploitation of the possibilities offered by histocompatibility haplotype analysis, population studies of JRA in the next decade might be expected to yield important information leading to the determination of its etiology.

REFERENCES

1. Glover, J.A. Milroy lectures of the incidence of rheumatic diseases. *Lancet*. 1:499–505, 1930.
2. Brewer, E.J., Bass, J., Baum, J. et al. Current proposed revision of JRA criteria. *Arthritis Rheum*. 20 (suppl):195–9, 1977.
3. Ansell, B.M. Juvenile chronic polyarthritis: Series 3. *Arthritis Rheum*. 20 (suppl):176–8, 1977.
4. Bywaters, E.G.L. Diagnostic Criteria for Still's Disease. Edited by P.H. Bennett and P.H. Wood. In *Population Studies of the Rheumatic Diseases*. New York: Excerpta Medica Foundation, 1968.
5. Baum, J. Epidemiology of juvenile rheumatoid arthritis (JRA). *Arthritis Rheum*. 20 (suppl):158–60, 1977.
6. Cassidy, J.T., (informal discussion). *Arthritis Rheum*. 20 (suppl):164, 1977.
7. Kanyerezi, B.R., Baddeley, H., and Kisumba, D. Rheumatoid arthritis in Ugandan Africans. *Ann Rheum Dis*. 29:616–21, 1970.
8. Laaksonen, A.-L. A prognostic study of juvenile rheumatoid arthritis. *Acta Paediatr Scand*. 166 (suppl):1966.
9. Sullivan, D.B., Cassidy, J.T., and Petty, R.E. Pathogenic implications of age of onset in juvenile rheumatoid arthritis. *Arthritis Rheum*. 18:251–5, 1975.
10. Hanson, V., Kornreich, H.K., Bernstein, B. et al. Three subtypes of juvenile rheumatoid arthritis. Correlations of age at onset, sex and serologic factors. *Arthritis Rheum*. 20 (suppl):184–6, 1977.
11. Hill, R. Juvenile arthritis in various racial groups in British Columbia. *Arthritis Rheum*. 20 (suppl):162, 1977.
12. Hill, R.H., and Robinson, H.S. Rheumatoid arthritis and ankylosing spondylitis in British Columbia Indians: their prevalence and the challenge of management. *Can Med Assoc J*. 100:509–11, 1969.
13. Stillman, J.S., and Barry, P.E. Juvenile rheumatoid arthritis: Series 2. *Arthritis Rheum*. 20 (suppl):171–5, 1977.
14. Ansell, B.M., and Bywaters, E.G.L. Rheumatoid arthritis (Still's disease). *Ped Clin N Amer*. 10:921–39, 1963.
15. Bywaters, E.G.L. Ankylosing spondylitis in childhood. *Clin Rheum Dis*. 2:387–96, 1976.
16. Ladd, J.R., Cassidy, J.T., and Martel, W. Juvenile ankylosing spondylitis. *Arthritis Rheum*. 14:579–90, 1971.

18

17. Schaller, J.G. Juvenile rheumatoid arthritis: Series 1. *Arthritis Rheum.* 20 (suppl):165–70, 1977.

18. Schaller, J.G., Smiley, W.K., and Ansell, B.M. Iridocyclitis of juvenile rheumatoid arthritis (JRA, Still's disease). *Arthritis Rheum.* 16:130, 1973.

19. Chylack, L.T. The ocular manifestations of juvenile rheumatoid arthritis. *Arthritis Rheum.* 20 (suppl):217–23, 1977.

20. Cassidy, J.T., Sullivan, D.B., and Petty, R.E. Clinical patterns of chronic iridocyclitis in children with juvenile rheumatoid arthritis. *Arthritis Rheum.* 20 (suppl):224–7, 1977.

21. Steere, A.C., Malawista, S.E., Syndman, D.R. et al. Lyme arthritis: an epidemic of oligoarticular arthritis in children and adults in three Connecticut communities. *Arthritis Rheum.* 20:7–17, 1977.

22. Cassidy, J.T., Shillis, J.L., and Brandon, F.B. Viral antibody titers to rubella and rubeola in JRA. *Pediatrics.* 54:239–44, 1974.

23. Ogra, P.L., Chiba, Y., Ogra, S.S. et al. Rubella virus infection in JRA. *Lancet.* 1:1157–61, 1975.

24. Phillips, P.E. Virologic studies in RA. *Rheumatology.* 6:353–60, 1975.

25. Ansell, B.M., Bywaters, E.G.L., and Lawrence, J.S. Familial aggregation and twin studies in Still's disease. *Rheumatology.* 2:37–61, 1969.

3 The Role of Infection in Arthritis

J. Roger Hollister

There are several compelling reasons for considering the possible role of infection in children with juvenile rheumatoid arthritis (JRA). First, a number of viral infections in children and adults may be associated with arthritis, usually of a self-limited nature, and often resemble the polyarticular character of rheumatoid arthritis. Second, children with JRA, in particular those with systemic disease, have fever, rash, and adenopathy which resemble the findings in many viral illnesses. In addition, this disease often has an explosive onset which suggests a viral illness. Third, although JRA is frequently considered an autoimmune disease, no putative antibodies to self-antigens have been described which prove a cause of the disease. Finally, the several extrahepatic manifestations of hepatitis-B virus (HBV) infection include arthritis, rashes, and disseminated organ system disease not dissimilar from JRA.

There are two sections to this chapter; the first describes the clinical features of viral infections which may produce arthritis and provides some differe..tial diagnostic information for evaluating a child with the acute onset of arthritis pointing out the suggestive information which clinically might link viral infection to JRA. In the second section of the chapter experimental information concerning recovery of viruses from patients with JRA or other indirect evidence of viral infection is reviewed. In addition, there is a summary of the experimental information which might lead to a hypothesis as to the mechanism by which an as yet undetected virus might cause the prolonged arthritis in JRA. From this information one might gain better insight into the future directions of investigation.

VIRAL ILLNESS WITH ARTHRITIS

Rubella virus can cause arthritis in two situations. In the first, there is a well-recognized polyarticular arthritis associated with natural infection with rubella. Secondly, immunization with attenuated rubella vaccine has produced arthritis with which the clinician should be familiar. An arthritis associated with natural rubella or German measles has been recognized at least since 1918 when Geiger described an epidemic of German measles occurring in a city next to an army training camp[1] in which 36 patients were reported to have arthritis with the infection. Subsequent studies of both epidemic and episodic rubella have recorded a frequency of arthritis as high as 15% in adults with rubella.[2-4] In general, arthritis begins within one to three days of the exanthem, which may be preceded by fever and malaise, is polyarticular, and most characteristically involves the small joints in the hands. Although self-limited, lasting five days to two weeks, it may be quite resistant to antiinflammatory treatment. The incidence of arthritis appears to be considerably higher in adults with infection than in children. On the other hand, the initial report of recovery of the rubella virus from the talonavicular joint occurred in a 14-month old child with rubella.[5] Once the acute episode of viral infection is over, there appear to be no residua. In follow-up studies of up to 10 years rubella arthritis does not appear to be a harbinger of rheumatoid arthritis.[6] An initial report of the seroconversion to rheumatoid factor positivity of patients with rubella has never been reproduced.[7] In fact the technique used was an inhibition assay prone to false positive results or interference by non–anti-IgG proteins. The patients who may demonstrate rheumatoid factor during acute illness do so probably as the result of antigenic challenge as is seen in a number of other diseases such as tuberculosis or subacute bacterial endocarditis.

Immunization with attenuated rubella vaccine causes different articular manifestations than infection with wild virus. Arthritis following immunization does not run a singular course but is prone to recurrences over a several month period.[8,9] Vaccine-induced arthritis most often affects the knees and is more prevalent with vaccines raised in dog kidney than with the duck or Cendehill vaccines.[10] Onset of joint swelling can be from a few days to up to 55 days following immunization, single episodes of arthritis lasting as long as 40 days. Of forty children with vaccine-induced arthritis recently studied, 11 had recurrent episodes lasting from one to five days.[9] The joints affected were the same as during the initial episode. The recurrences tended to become less frequent and milder with passage of time and long-term prognosis after three years of follow-up appears to be very favorable. The immunization program has not produced more cases of JRA than would have been seen in an unvaccinated population. As with streptococcal infection, trauma, and stress, immunization can be viewed as a trigger for the clinical expression of JRA whose cause as yet remains unknown.

The mechanism of vaccine-induced arthritis appears to be similar to the natural disease. Ogra and Herd have recovered rubella vaccine virus from joints undergoing a recurrent synovitis for as long as three to four months following vaccination.[11] Antibody to rubella appeared in the synovial fluid at the same time. Studies of the host's immune response to rubella vaccination have failed to find differences in antibody levels between those that developed arthritis and those that did not.

A final bit of experimental information suggests that rubella virus has an unusual affinity for immature chondrocytes in the cartilage of experimental animals.[12] Viral infection or retention on the surface of cartilage will be described subsequently when possible mechanisms for the role of infection in JRA are discussed.

Clinicians should be aware that although the duck embryo or Cendehill strains of virus are used for vaccination now, there is still a considerable incidence of both polyarticular and monoarticular arthritis following vaccination. A careful history, particularly of patients presenting with knee arthritis, should be obtained if rubella vaccination occurred within two months of the arthritis onset. In patients who experience vaccine-induced arthritis, recurrences may be expected, but they tend to be milder than the initial episode, and the ultimate prognosis is extremely favorable.

Experimental information concerning the role of rubella in JRA has not succeeded in showing a link between virus and JRA but serves to illustrate the approaches which have been taken. A provocative report by Grazell and Beck indicated that although rheumatoid synovial cells in culture could be infected with a variety of viruses, they were not capable of supporting rubella replication.[13] The implication was that a preexistent rubella infection of these cells led to specific interference of further rubella infectivity. The rubella virus did appear to penetrate the cultured cells, and resistance was not due to production of interferon. Subsequent studies have failed to reproduce these results, and rheumatoid cells do in fact appear to be able to support rubella replication.[14] The mechanism for rheumatoid cell resistance, if it exists, may be related to increased production of hyaluronic acid by the rheumatoid synovial cells in culture.[15] It has been shown that hyaluronic acid added to cultures of normal synovial cells inhibits replication of rubella. In addition, hyaluronidase treatment of rheumatoid cells allowed infection of these cells. Whether such an explanation applied to the original report is not certain because hyaluronic acid apparently does interfere with viral attachment to the cell.

Stimulated by the initial report of rheumatoid synovial cell resistance, several authors have used the rubella antibody response in JRA patients to link virus and rheumatoid disease indirectly.[16,17] Evidence suggests either that children with JRA do not have extraordinary titers against rubella virus or that the elevations can be explained by a generalized hypergammaglobulinemia. Therefore, the response to rubella is part of a generalized hyperresponsiveness in humoral immunity demonstrated in these patients. A single report of the identification of rubella virus antigen in the synovial fluids of patients with JRA has not been corroborated.[18]

In the past six years there has been impressive proof demonstrating that hepatitis-B virus (formerly known as Australia antigen hepatitis) can be associated with symptoms of a variety of collagen vascular diseases. These manifestations have both practical and theoretical interest. The first descriptions were of a serum sicknesslike illness preceding icteric hepatitis associated with HBV.[19-22] These patients have a multiorgan disease including rashes which are often urticarial, arthritis of a polyarticular nature, fever, and nephritis. These symptoms are usually of short duration, approximately 7 to 14 days, but may precede the development of jaundice and overt hepatitis by as much as six weeks. The arthritis is self-limited and without residua.

The mechanism for development of these extrahepatic manifestations has been successfully investigated. Significant immunopathologic events predicted from experimental immune complex models have been found in the prodromal HBV illness. In the prodromal phase, the surface protein antigen of HBV is demonstrable in serum and synovial fluid of patients with coincident lowering of complement levels in both serum and synovial fluid.[19,20] With the onset of icteric hepatitis, prodromal symptoms including arthritis wane, the complement returns to normal, and one can demonstrate the presence of antibody to HBV.

Patients who demonstrate arthritis in the prodromal phase seem to differ in their immune response when compared to those who do not. Those suffering the serum sicknesslike picture tend to form an IgG_1, an IgG_3, and IgM response to the antigen.[23] Circulating immune complexes of HBV antigen and these immunoglobulins exist in the cryoprecipitates from the serum of patients with prodroma but not those with uncomplicated hepatitis. There is in vitro evidence that immune complexes of HBV antigen and specific antibody are capable of fixing complement by both classical and alternative pathways, thus the mechanism for the clinical sequence seems well established. Following viremia with HBV the host responds with specific antibody, and immune complexes are formed which deposit in skin, joint fluid, and kidneys, invoking inflammation and multiorgan symptomatology. Following this phase of antigen excess, the immune response produces antibody excess with rapid elimination of circulating immune complexes and a resolution of prodromal symptoms and signs. Thereafter the hepatic, icteric phases ensue.

The association of HBV and periarteritis nodosa (PAN) provides a different example of viral infection and host immune response. Between 30% and 40% of patients with PAN have chronic HBV viremia demonstrable in their serum.[24-26] In the acute phase it is possible to demonstrate HBV antigen, immunoglobulin, and complement in the blood vessels of affected organs. Most of these patients also demonstrate increased hepatic involvement with their disease compared to patients who do not chronically carry HBV. Although an etiologic link between viremia and PAN is only inferential, chronic carrying of this virus appears to segregate a subset of patients who may have a better prognosis than those that do not.[26] It is not clear whether failure by the host to make an appropriate antibody response to this virus and thereby clear it from serum is responsible for the symptomatology. An alternative explanation might reason that these patients have a defective immune response as part of their periarteritis nodosa which then leads to ineffective removal of a pathologically insignificant virus.

Despite the provocative information concerning HBV in periarteritis nodosa, other diseases such as rheumatoid arthritis appear to have no relationship to this particular virus. Numerous studies have sought the demonstration of HBV antigen and/or antibody in patients with rheumatoid arthritis by sensitive techniques but there is no greater incidence of either in these patients than in normal controls.[27,28]

The third association is between HBV and chronic membranoproliferative glomerulonephritis.[22] There have been reports both in adults and children of demonstration of HBV in renal biopsies of patients with chronic glomerulonephritis. The host response and the relationship to pathophysiology in these patients is not yet defined. Again the information is only inferential and cannot currently sort out cause from effect, but further studies may clarify the issue.

Various disease associations with HBV can supply the clinician with diagnostic information and can provide the investigator with stimulating leads. Different clinical expressions of HBV may relate to an altered immune response by the host rather than differences in the virus. The dissimilar clinical patterns of JRA (systemic, polyarticular, or pauciarticular) may represent a similar diversity in symptomatology due to host variance and not disease difference.

Other viral associations with arthritis fall into two groups: those that are reported infrequently with common childhood diseases, and viral epidemics not common to the United States but illustrative of some situations similar to the recently described Lyme arthritis. Mumps,[29-31] infectious mononucleosis,[32] chicken pox,[33] and erythema infectiosum[34] have all had cases described with concurrent arthritis. The arthritides are self-limited pains and swellings of one or several joints lasting at most for a few days. No residua have been noted to any of these, and the illnesses have not appeared to lead to development of JRA. In general arthritis follows other manifestations of the viral syndrome including the rash of chicken pox and thus should provide no particular diagnostic confusion. On the other hand, arthritis associated with mumps, which has been known for over a hundred years, may in fact precede the development of parotitis and most of the described cases have been reported with coexistent orchitis.[29,30] No studies of viral isolation or other techniques to understand the pathogenesis of these arthritides have been performed.

In other parts of the world, viruses such as that responsible for Chikungunya or dengue fever or smallpox are capable of causing considerable morbidity from the associated arthritis.[35] For physicians practicing in these areas the association probably produces little diagnostic confusion and they do provide illustrative examples of viral illnesses and arthritis that can spread through a community. Lyme arthritis in the United States represents such a situation.

Lyme arthritis occurred in epidemic form in communities in Connecticut and serves as a prototype for investigators and clinicians alike.[36] Recognition of this new epidemic syndrome came about when four of 12 children in a small neighborhood were misdiagnosed as having JRA and another family reported that the mother, father, and two siblings all had arthritis. In the course of four years in these communities 51 patients, of which 39 were children, were identified as having a unique monoarticular or pauciarticular form of arthritis involving large joints. The episodes of synovitis lasted an average of one week, and the patients had a mean of three recurrences over one to several years. In 25% of the cases arthritis was preceded by an extraordinary rash which began as a papule and spread into a large erythematous lesion frequently measuring 20 to 50 mm in diameter. It tended to precede the joint swelling by approximately four weeks and was often accompanied by fever and headache. The rash seemed connected etiologically to the arthritis in that only two residents of the community who had the rash did not go on to develop arthritis as well.

Further studies in the epidemiology of this new arthritis showed that the peak incidence occurred in the summer, but in some families and close neighbors new cases occurred one to two years apart. Only two individuals were HLA-B27 positive, and other extensive bacteriologic, virologic, and serologic tests were negative including serologic evidence for arbor virus infection such as is believed to be the causative agent in the Ross River epidemic arthritis in Australia.[37] However, some studies indicated that patients had cryoprecipitates in their serum during the rash and arthritis. This new form of arthritis had attacks of short duration, followed by recurrences with complete remissions in between. The patients did not have antinuclear antibodies, there was no iridocyclitis, and some of the patients had lowered values of C3. In addition, the unique rash and presence of cryoprecipitates in the serum served to distinguish this arthritis from JRA, natural or vaccine rubella arthritis, or other transient nonrecurring synovitis in childhood.

Although the epidemiology of this arthritis suggests insect transmission, a vector has yet to be identified. It is also unclear if cases will remain confined to this geographic area; with modern transportation and a highly mobile population, cases outside Connecticut are likely to exist in the future. Unfortunately the considerable effort expended to

Table 1
Viral Infections Causing Arthritis

Common	Rubella-wild and vaccine
	Hepatitis B
	Mumps
	Varicella
	Infectious mononucleosis
	Erythema infectiosum
Epidemic	? Lyme arthritis
	Ross River
	Smallpox
Unknown	Transient synovitis

investigate Lyme arthritis is not likely to shed light on the patients frequently seen with transient synovitis with no particularly distinguishing features. The latter group of patients have swollen joints for one to several weeks with few other symptoms. Before the diagnostic interval of three months for JRA has passed the synovitis has fully resolved, recurrences and sequelae are not observed, and the children return to good health.

EXPERIMENTAL INFORMATION ON VIRUSES AND JRA

When evaluating the experimental approaches taken to investigate infectious origin of rheumatoid arthritis, one must note that although as yet no single etiologic agent has been discovered there continue to be creative approaches to the problem as technology in infectious disease improves. Attempts at uncovering an infectious agent have been under way for more than 50 years but the lack of positive results should not discourage one from pursuing this goal. Although rheumatoid arthritis is currently viewed as autoimmune disease, an autoantigen has not been found, and it remains a viable alternative that an infection is either the trigger or the non–self-stimulus for the prolonged inflammatory response.

Direct isolation of an infective organism was the first method undertaken to find an infectious etiology. Beginning with attempts in the 1930s to culture bacteria from rheumatoid synovia and synovial fluid, these studies have become increasingly more sophisticated in their approaches.[38] With the inability to culture bacteria from these tissues investigators sought other organisms such as mycoplasma, diphtheroids, chlamydia, and finally viruses, by direct culture technique. Initial enthusiastic reports of mycoplasma isolation have not been confirmed by other laboratories.[39] The problem of contamination of specimens within a given laboratory remains an unresolved difficulty, for despite inclusion of control specimens from other diseases, one cannot eliminate the possibility that specimens from rheumatoid patients are more easily contaminated than those of other disease groups.

Techniques for implicating a viral infection have gone beyond the inoculation of specimens from rheumatoids into tissue culture. Recent attempts have included cell fusion, cocultivation, radioactive precursor incorporation, and assays of reverse transcriptase.[40,41] As yet these methods have produced uniformly negative results.

The electron microscope has been used to attempt to provide morphologic evidence of infection. Changes seen in rheumatoid tissue bear certain similarities to cells which have been transformed by virus infection. However, direct ultrastructural evidence of viral particles has not been possible.[42] Immunofluorescent attempts with specific antibodies directed against known viruses have been negative with the exception of an unconfirmed report of rubella antigen occurring in the synovial fluid sediment of patients with JRA.[18]

Antibody levels in serum and synovial fluid have been assayed as an indirect evidence of previous or ongoing infection with known viruses. By and large these studies have either shown normal antibody levels or elevations against several viruses suggesting a hyperactive response by the human host rather than specific viral causation.[40]

Recent investigations of the immunogenetics of patients with other forms of arthritis have offered exciting approaches to future studies of rheumatoid arthritis. Patients with ankylosing spondylitis, Reiter's syndrome and *Yersinia* arthritis all share a common histocompatibility antigen, HLA-B27. The incidence of this antigen in patients with these diseases is approximately 20 times higher than in the normal population. On the other hand, not all individuals carrying the HLA-B27 antigen are destined to develop arthritis although it appears that expression of this antigen puts the individual at an increased risk should one encounter the proper environmental stimulus. The example of the reactive arthritis following *Yersinia* infection provides a good illustration.[43] *Yersinia enterocolitica* is a gram-negative coliform bacterium which causes epidemic dysentery, particularly prevalent in Finland and the Scandinavian countries. Following the acute period of diarrhea there is a symptom-free interval and then onset of acute polyarthritis involving mainly large joints and joints of the lower extremities. Although the disease is usually self-limited some rather severe and prolonged disability can result. Population studies have indicated that most individuals may be susceptible to the dysenteric part of the illness, but only those individuals carrying HLA-B27 antigen have developed reactive arthritis. The occurrence of an epidemic of Reiter's syndrome following a *Shigella* outbreak on a Naval ship has provided another example. Years later the patients who developed reactive arthritis to this dysenteric organism were also found to be carriers of HLA-B27 antigen.[44] The results of these and other studies indicate that the gene responsible for HLA-B27 antigen expression is not directly causative of the illness but rather sets the stage for the development of arthritis following exposure to an infectious agent. Similar studies of histocompatibility antigens in patients with JRA and rheumatoid arthritis have failed to segregate a particular antigen with these diseases.[45,46] On the other hand, a recent report of increased frequency of Cw3 and Dw4 antigens in patients with rheumatoid arthritis indicates that there may be other genetic codes for the immune response.[47,48] The possibility still remains that clinical expression of rheumatoid arthritis will depend both on genetic constitution of the individual and on exposure to the environment, including a variety of infectious organisms (see Chapter 8).

Another experimental approach taken by several investigators has been the search for pathogenic material in rheumatoid patients in locations other than synovial tissue and fluid. From work in experimental animals it appears that models simulating rheumatoid arthritis with development of pathologic features of the human disease are caused by prolonged retention of phlogistic material on cartilage in the hard tissue within the joints of these animals.[49] Using antigens which could represent viral or bacterial products prolonged arthritis is induced in these animals through formation of tissue-bound immune complexes of specific antigen and antibody onto the cartilage surfaces of ligaments, menisci, and bone. These immune complexes exist for extraordinary lengths of time and appear to be outside the normal clearance mechanisms of the host. Supportive immunofluorescent data from humans with rheumatoid arthritis have indicated the deposition of immunoglobulin and complement components in the same areas within human tissue.[50] With recovery techniques developed in these experimental animals, it should be possible to search in the same sequestered locations in surgical specimens from humans with rheumatoid arthritis to uncover possible infectious agents bound to these tissues.

In conclusion, one might ask why the attempts to prove an infectious origin of JRA have failed. There are several reasonable explanations. The first is that of technology. In the past fifty years the science of organism detection has progressed significantly as evidenced by development of viral vaccines, the revelation of slow virus infections, and recovery of the bacillus responsible for Legionnaire's disease. Technologies of the future should continue to be applied to the study of JRA. The second explanation is that JRA is not caused by a unique infectious agent. Studies of patients with axial arthropathies and reactive arthritis suggest that individuals with susceptible genetic constitutions may respond with similar arthritis to several organisms such as *Yersinia* or *Shigella*. Infection may be a nonspecific stimulus by common or esoteric agents for a chronic stereotyped arthritic response by a genetically prone host. Rapid advancements in animal and human immunogenetics in the past decade have offered new tools for future study of JRA.

A final possible explanation is a combination of the first two. Studies of the prodrome of HBV hepatitis have shown that only part of the virus, the protein coat, is responsible for stimulating a response in the host for circulating immune complex disease. In experimental arthritis studies, antigens of low molecular weight similar to a fragment of a virus can cause prolonged inflammation if they cannot be cleared by the host. Therefore, future investigations should utilize new technologies in infectious disease and the fast-expanding information of immunogenetics and host defense mechanisms to probe further the role of infection in JRA.

REFERENCES

1. Geiger, J.C. Epidemic of German measles in a city adjacent to an Army cantonment and its probable relation thereto. *JAMA.* 70:1818–30, 1918.

2. Fry, J., Dillane, J.B., and Fry, L. Rubella, 1962. *Br Med J.* 2:833–4, 1962.

3. Phillips, C.A., Behbehani, A.M., Johnson, L.W., and Melnick, J.L. Isolation of rubella virus: an epidemic characterized by rash and arthritis. *JAMA.* 191:615–18, 1965.

4. Brody, J.A., Sever, J.L., McAllister, R. et al. Rubella epidemic on St. Paul Island in the Pribilofs, 1963. I. Epidemiologic, clinical and serologic findings. *JAMA.* 191:619–23, 1965.

5. Hildebrandt, H.M., and Maassab, H.F. Rubella synovitis in a one-year-old patient. *N Engl J Med.* 274:1428–30, 1966.

6. Kantor, T.G., and Tanner, M. Rubella arthritis and rheumatoid arthritis. *Arthritis Rheum.* 5:378–83, 1962.

7. Johnson, R.E., and Hall, A.P. Rubella arthritis: report of cases studied by latex tests. *N Engl J Med.* 258:743–5, 1958.

8. Spruance, S.L., Klock, L.E., Bailey, A. et al. Recurrent joint symptoms in children vaccinated with HPV-77 DK12 rubella vaccine. *J Pediatr.* 80:413–17, 1972.

9. Thompson, G.R., Weiss, J.J., Eloise, M.I. et al. Intermittent arthritis following rubella vaccination: a three year follow-up. *Am J Dis Child.* 125:526–30, 1973.

10. Austin, S.M., Altman, R., Barnes, E.K., and Dougherty, W.J. Joint reactions in children vaccinated against rubella. Study I. Comparison of two vaccines. Study II. Comparison of three vaccines. *Am J Epidemiol.* 95:53–8, 59–66, 1972.

11. Ogra, P.L., and Herd, J.K. Arthritis associated with induced rubella infection. *J Immunol.* 107:810–13, 1971.

12. London, W.T., Fuccillo, D.A., Anderson, B., and Sever, J.L. Concentration of rubella virus antigen in chondrocytes of congenitally infected rabbits. *Nature.* (London) 226:172–3, 1970.

13. Grayzel, A.I., and Beck, C. Rubella infection of synovial cells and the resistance of cells derived from patients with rheumatoid arthritis. *J Exp Med.* 131:367–73, 1970.

14. Anderson, C.H. Replication of viruses in cultured JRA synovial cells, abstracted. *Arthritis Rheum.* 16:114, 1973.

15. Patterson, R.L., Peterson, D.A., Deinhardt, F., and Howard, F. Rubella and rheumatoid arthritis: hyaluronic acid and susceptibility of cultured rheumatoid synovial cells to viruses. *Proc Soc Exp Biol Med.* 149:594–8, 1975.

16. Cassidy, J.T., Shillis, J.L., Brandon, F.B. et al. Viral antibody titres to rubella and rubeola in juvenile rheumatoid arthritis. *Pediatrics.* 54:239–44, 1974.

17. Linnemann, C.C., Levinson, J.E., Buncher, C.R., and Schiff, G.M. Rubella antibody titres in juvenile rheumatoid arthritis. *Ann Rheum Dis.* 34:354–8, 1975.

18. Ogra, P.L., Ogra, S.S., Chiba, Y. et al. Rubella virus infection in juvenile rheumatoid arthritis. *Lancet.* 1:1157–61, 1975.

19. Onion, D.K., Crumpacker, C.D., and Gilliland, B.C. Arthritis of hepatitis associated with Australia antigen. *Ann Int Med.* 75:29–33, 1971.

20. Alpert, E., Isselbacher, K.J., and Schur, P.H. The pathogenesis of arthritis associated with viral hepatitis. Complement component studies. *N Engl J Med.* 285:185–9, 1971.

21. Segool, R.A., Lejtenyi, C., and Taussig, L.M. Articular and cutaneous manifestations of viral hepatitis. *J Pediatr.* 87:709–12, 1975.

22. Gocke, D.J. Extrahepatic manifestations of viral hepatitis. *Am J Med Sci.* 270:49–52, 1975.

23. Wands, J.R., Mann, E., Alpert, E., and Isselbacher, K.J. The pathogenesis of arthritis associated with acute hepatitis-B surface antigen-positive hepatitis. *J Clin Invest.* 55:930–6, 1975.

24. Gocke, D.J., Hsu, K., Morgan, C. et al. Association between polyarteritis and Australia antigen. *Lancet.* 2:1149–53, 1970.

25. Trepo, C.G., Thivolet, J., and Prince, A.M. Australia antigen and polyarteritis nodosa. *Am J Dis Child.* 123:390–92, 1972.

26. Sergent, J.S., and Christian, C.L. Necrotizing vasculitis after acute serous otitis media. *Ann Int Med.* 81:195–9, 1974.

27. Panush, R.S., Alpert, E., and Schur, P.H. Absence of Au antigen and antibody in patients with rheumatic disease. *Arthritis Rheum.* 14:782–3, 1971.

28. Marcolango, R., and Debolini, A. Incidence of hepatitis associated antigen HAA and homologous antibody in patients with rheumatoid arthritis. *Vox Sang.* 28:9–18, 1975.

29. Applebaum, F., Kohn, J., Steinman, R.E., and Stearn, M.A. Mumps arthritis. *Arch Int Med.* (Chicago) 90:217–23, 1952.

30. Lass, R., and Shephard, E. Mumps arthritis. *Br Med J.* 2:1613–14, 1961.

31. Gold, H.E., Boxerbaum, B., and Leslie, H.J. Mumps arthritis. *Am J Dis Child.* 116:547–8, 1968.

32. Adebonigo, F.O. Monoarticular arthritis: an unusual manifestation of infectious mononucleosis. *Clin Pediatr.* 11:549–50, 1972.

33. Friedman, A., and Naveh, Y. Polyarthritis associated with chicken pox. *Am J Dis Child.* 122:179–80, 1971.

34. Ager, E.A., Chin, T.D.Y., and Poland, J.D. Epidemic erythema infectiosum. *N Engl J Med.* 275:1326–31, 1966.

35. Smith, J.W., and Sanford, J.P. Viral arthritis. *Ann Int Med.* 67:651–9, 1967.

36. Steere, A.C., Malawista, S.E., Syndman, D.R. et al. Lyme arthritis. *Arthritis Rheum.* 20:7–17, 1977.

37. Clarke, J.A., Marshall, I.D., and Gard, G. Annually recurrent epidemic polyarthritis and Ross River virus activity in a coastal area of New South Wales. I. Occurrence of the disease. II. Mosquitoes, viruses and wildlife. *Am J Trop Med Hyg.* 22:543, 551–68, 1973.

38. Dawson, M.H., Olmstead, M., and Boots, R.H. Bacteriologic investigations on the blood, synovial fluid and subcutaneous nodules in rheumatoid (chronic infectious) arthritis. *Arch Int Med.* 49:173–80, 1932.

39. Middleton, P.J., and Highton, T.C. Failure to show mycoplasmas and cytopathogenic virus in rheumatoid arthritis. *Ann Rheum Dis.* 34:369–72, 1975.

40. Phillips, P.E. Virologic studies in rheumatoid arthritis. *Rheumatology.* (Basel) 6:353–60, 1976.

41. Spruance, S.L., Richards, O.C., Smith, C.B., and Ward, J.R. DNA polymerase activity of cultured rheumatoid synovial cells. *Arthritis Rheum.* 18:229–35, 1975.

42. Wynne-Roberts, C.R., and Anderson, C.L. Light and electron microscopic comparison of juvenile normal and rheumatoid synovium, abstracted. *J Rheumatol.* 1 (suppl 1):80, 1974.

43. Aho, K., Ahvonen, P., Lassas, A. et al. HLA antigen-27 and reactive arthritis. *Lancet.* 2:157, 1973.

44. Calin, A., and Fries, J.F. Epidemic Reiter's syndrome. Genetics and environment. *Arthritis Rheum.* 18:390–91, 1975.

45. Gibson, D.J., Carpenter, C.B., and Stillman, J.S. Reexamination of histocompatibility antigens found in patients with juvenile rheumatoid arthritis. *N Engl J Med.* 293:636–8, 1975.

46. Schaller, J.G., Ochs, H.D., Thomas, E.D. et al. Histocompatibility antigens in childhood-onset arthritis. *J Pediatr.* 88:926–30, 1976.

47. Stastny, P. Mixed lymphocyte culture typing cells from patients with rheumatoid arthritis. *Tissue Antigens.* 4:571, 1974.

48. McMichael, A.J., Sasazuki, T., McDevitt, H.O., and Payne, R.O. Increased frequency of HLA-Cw3 and HLA-Dw4 in rheumatoid arthritis. *Arthritis Rheum.* 20:1037–42, 1977.

49. Hollister, J.R., and Mannik, M. Antigen retention in joint tissues in antigen-induced synovitis. *Clin Exp Immunol.* 16:615–27, 1974.

50. Cooke, T.D., Hurd, E.R., Bienenstock, J. et al. The immunofluorescent identification of immunoglobulins and complement in rheumatoid articular collagenous tissue, abstracted. *Arthritis Rheum.* 15:433, 1972.

4 Immunological Abnormalities in Juvenile Rheumatoid Arthritis

John J. Miller III

There are no immunologic abnormalities yet recognized which are unique to juvenile rheumatoid arthritis (JRA). A large number of nonspecific immunologic or serum protein changes have been described, including elevated sedimentation rates, increased serum concentrations of immunoglobulins, C3, and C-reactive protein. In a few of the severe systemic-onset patients the hyperglobulinemia can be as severe as in serum sickness, and plasma cells are occasionally seen in the blood of these extreme cases. None of these findings is helpful diagnostically, but when present, they are helpful in following the course of the disease in an individual patient.

The search for more specific and diagnostic abnormalities and for potential pathogenic mechanisms has paralleled the developing knowledge of adult-onset rheumatoid arthritis. The greatest efforts have been in trying to discover a corollary to adult rheumatoid factor (RF) and in exploring the incidence and meaning of the presence of antinuclear antibodies (ANA). Less work has been done to examine directly the role of immune complexes or the role of thymus-derived (T) lymphocytes and delayed hypersensitivity.

RHEUMATOID FACTOR

Rheumatoid factor is an IgM antibody to IgG first discovered as a complex in sera of adults with rheumatoid arthritis. The antibody has a relatively weak affinity for native globulin and it can be easily demonstrated by its ability to agglutinate globulin-coated particles such as red cells or latex particles. There are several red cell agglutination techniques which vary in sensitivity. The latex fixation (LF) test is less selective than the red cell tests but currently is most widely used.

The first study of children with JRA was reported by Bywaters, Carter and Scott from England using one of the more specific red cell agglutination techniques.[1] They studied 142 children who had been followed for periods from four to eight years and found a very low incidence of positive tests compared to that in adults. The incidence was lowest in those children with onset under the age of four years and increased with age of onset. Sera from individual patients usually remained negative if they were negative at onset, but changes occurred from negative to transiently positive to permanently positive, or from positive to negative in about half the patients. The persistence of rheumatoid factor usually was associated with persistent disease activity. Similar results were reported by Laaksonen in a larger study from Finland.[2]

The incidence of positive LF tests was studied by Laaksonen, Cassidy and Valkenburg,[3] and Hanson, Drexler and Kornreich.[4] All these groups found a higher incidence of positive LF tests than of red cell agglutination tests, higher incidence of LF positivity with increasing age of onset (Figure 1), a relative stability of test results in individual children with time, an association of LF positivity with more persistent and severe disease, and a lack of selectivity of positive LF tests for JRA. Positive tests were also seen in systemic lupus erythematosus (SLE), scleroderma, chronic liver disease, lymphomas, dermatomyositis and subacute bacterial endocarditis.

It is reasonably certain that a major part of the pathogenesis of joint inflammation in adult rheumatoid arthritis results from activation of the complement system by IgM rheumatoid factor bound to its antigen, IgG. The absence of IgM rheumatoid factor in most children with JRA has led to a search for other forms of antiglobulin antibody which might have a similar role. Torrigiani, Ansell, Chown and Roitt used an immunoadsorption method to study sera from children with active and inactive JRA and from normal children.[5] In this method normal pooled globulin was made insoluble by bis-diazotization. The insoluble globulin was mixed with the serum to be tested, washed, and then exposed to a mild acid buffer. Mild acid breaks antigen-antibody bonds. Immunoglobulins released by the acid buffer could be measured and were assumed to be antiglobulin antibodies, in other words, to be rheumatoid factors whether of IgM, IgG, or IgA types. Normal children were found to have measurable IgG antiglobulins by this method but children with active JRA had distinctly greater concentrations; the children with inactive JRA usually had concentrations in the normal range. This particular method has not been widely used, but elevated IgG antiglobulin concentrations have been reported in JRA using other methods. Florin-Christensen et al. made globulin insoluble by binding it to betonite particles and then using the particles in a manner similar to the bis-diazotized globulin.[6] They found no antiglobulin activity in normal children or adults but found some in 48 of 50

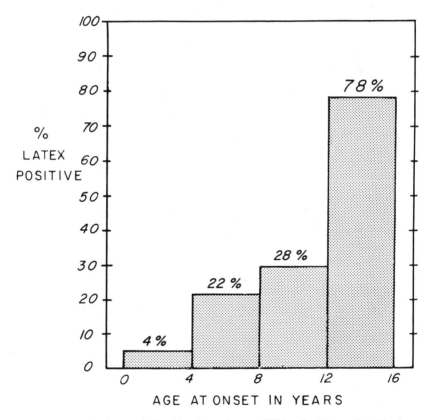

Figure 1.   Graph shows relationship of age of onset of JRA to incidence of positive latex fixation reactions by euglobulin fraction of serum, a particularly sensitive test positive in 95% of adults with RA.[4]

Reproduced with permission from the author, Victor Hanson, M.D., and the publisher, Grune and Stratton, Inc., from: Hanson, Drexler, and Kornreich. The relationship of rheumatoid factor to age of onset in juvenile rheumatoid arthritis. *Arthritis and Rheumatism.* 12:83, 1969.

children or young adults with JRA. In most cases the concentrations were low and there was no difference between sera from patients with active or inactive disease. The most extensive study of this sort is that of Bianco, Panush, Stillman and Schur.[7] Globulin was made insoluble by glutaraldehyde which was then used as described above. Presumed antiglobulin antibodies of IgM, IgA, and IgG type were found in sera from normal adults and from children with JRA. The mean concentrations of IgG antiglobulins were significantly greater in the children but there was a wide range and many individual values were within the adult normal range. Usually there was a good correlation between the presence of IgM antiglobulins and IgG and IgA antiglobulins but in some patients only elevated IgG and IgA antiglobulins were found, in synovial fluid as well as in serum. Children with antiglobulins of all three types had the most severe disease. The authors did not describe the clinical condition of those children with elevated levels of IgG and IgA antiglobulins in the absence of IgM antiglobulins.

In a later paper, Bianco, Dobkin and Schur described an alternative method of isolating IgG rheumatoid factors using globulins covalently bound to Sepharose in a chromatography column.[8] Sera from four patients with JRA were studied. Again, the absolute amount of IgG antiglobulin in these sera was within a range isolated from normal sera. However, for the first time it was shown that the IgG antiglobulins from the patients with JRA could fix complement, a necessary feature if these antibodies have a pathogenic role. IgG antiglobulins from normal persons did not fix complement.

Another species of antiglobulin, pepsin agglutinator, was studied by Munthe.[9] When globulin is digested by pepsin antigenic sites become available which react with antibodies present in sera from a large proportion of normal adults. In this study these pepsin agglutinators were found in sera from 44% of normal children, in sera from 55% of children with JRA under 15 years of age, and in 83% of children with JRA older than 15 years. These figures compared to an incidence of 12% positive LF tests in the group studied. These specialized forms of antiglobulins were resistant to reduction by 2-mercaptoethanol and were therefore thought to be IgG. A pathogenic role for pepsin agglutinators is highly speculative, however.

More pertinent may be Munthe's study of plasma cells in the synovial tissue of actively involved children with JRA.[10] Using fluorescent techniques he showed that all immunoglobulin classes and all the subclasses of IgG were being produced in the diseased synovial tissue. IgG_1-, IgG_2-, and IgG_3-producing cells predominated. None of the plasma cells in frozen sections bound aggregated globulin, a test for classical rheumatoid factor. However, after mild treatment with pepsin many of the plasma cells did bind globulin, a fact interpreted as demonstrating "hidden" IgG rheumatoid factors. Some cells had pepsin agglutinators. Complement products were deposited in these tissues suggesting that binding to locally deposited complexes was taking place.

In my laboratory an attempt to duplicate Bianco et al.'s[7] method with glutaraldehyde-treated globulin was unsuccessful because large amounts of nonspecific protein bound to our reagent.[11] However, comparison with several other forms of globulin immunoadsorbents showed that Bianco et al.'s[8] second method using chromatography columns of Sepharose-bound globulin was quite specific in extracting immunoglobulins which could often be shown to have LF activity even when the tested sera had been LF negative.[11] As in earlier studies, some activity was found in normal children. None of the 13 children with pauciarticular-onset JRA had concentrations of antiglobulins greater than those found in normal children even though three had low titers of LF activity. Eleven of 39 children with polyarticular-onset or systemic-onset JRA had antiglobulin concentrations greater than two standard deviations from the mean of concentrations in sera from normal children, but only four of these 11 had LF-negative sera at the time of testing so this method did not reveal a large proportion of children with IgG antiglobulin activity.

IgM antiglobulins may be present but specifically bound to autologous IgG and therefore not available to agglutinate heterologous IgG-coated particles. This possibility was studied in children with JRA by Moore, Dorner and Zuckner.[12] Sera were acidified to break antigen-antibody bonds and then run through a Sephadex chromatography column which separated IgM from IgG by size. The IgM fractions of six of 13 LF-negative sera were LF-positive when separated from autologous IgG by this method. IgG fractions were not positive, as might have been expected if IgG antiglobulins were present. The only clinical parameters which stood out in the six children with these "occult" IgM antiglobulins were earlier age of onset and longer duration of disease. This seems surprising since easily detected IgM antiglobulins have a higher incidence in older children and the incidence changes little with time.[1-4] However, Moore (personal communication) has extended these studies and has found up to 60% of children with JRA have IgM fractions which fix complement to IgG-coated red blood cells when separated in this manner.

Thus there are enough data to conclude that children with elevated levels of IgM antiglobulins have the worst prognoses.[1-4,8] The significance of elevated concentrations of IgG or IgA antiglobulins is not clear. The possibility that classical IgM rheumatoid factors are present

SEPHAROSE – FII

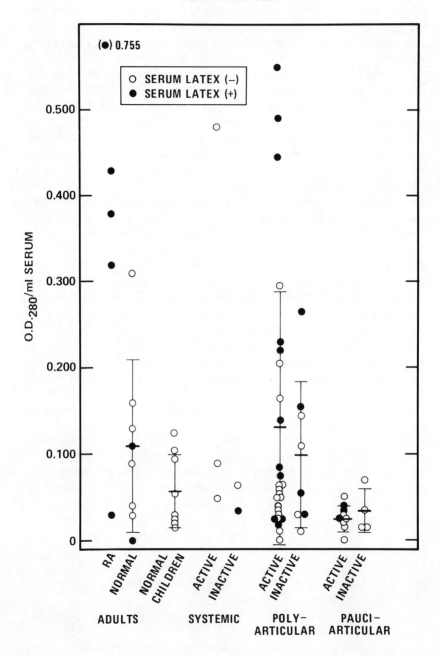

in many children with JRA but are masked by combination with IgG, presumably with a high affinity, remains unconfirmed. Since IgG antiglobulins seem to be present in normal children as well as those with JRA it will be necessary to demonstrate a significant difference in function of those found in JRA if they are to be assigned a pathogenic role. An important distinction would be the possibility that IgG antiglobulins from children with JRA can fix complement while those from normal children cannot, but this needs to be demonstrated in a large study.[8]

ANTINUCLEAR ANTIBODIES

The currently used fluorescent antibody tests for antinuclear factors were originally expected to be quick tests for the presence of the LE cell factor and thus diagnostic of systemic lupus erythematosus (SLE). They are performed by exposing naked nuclei on a section or smear to the test serum and then looking for the presence of attached globulin, assumed to be specific antibody, with a fluorescent anti-human globulin antibody. It soon became apparent that this method was quite nonspecific and that positive tests were found in many diseases including JRA.[13-15]

It is not possible to cite absolute figures for incidence of ANA in JRA because there has been no standardization of substrate and because varied titers have been used to define negative from positive. The latter practice has developed because normal persons develop an increasing incidence of low titers of ANA with age, and arbitrary cutoff titers are needed to distinguish normal adults from those with disease. Human granulocyte nuclei bind ANA with a higher incidence from children with JRA than do nuclei from other species or tissues.[16] In my experience this substrate will result in positive reactions with only 5% of undiluted sera from children with nonrheumatic disease, and I therefore believe *any* positive test in children is worthy of interest.

Despite differences in methods some correlations between clinical condition and positive tests for ANA are universally accepted. The first

---

Figure 2. Scattergram shows values of protein measured as OD_{280} per milliliter of applied sera eluted by acid from columns of globulin-coated Sepharose after passage of test sera.[11] Protein eluted was IgG with varying proportions of IgA and IgM. Mean and standard deviations are shown when adequate numbers of observations are available. Highest values among children are in active, polyarticular JRA, with overlap between normal children and all JRA groups. Only 4 with latex (–) JRA in this study had levels of elutable protein greater than 2 standard deviations above mean found in normal children.

Reprinted with permission from the publisher, The Arthritis Foundation, from Miller, Olds-Arroyo, and Akasaka. Antiglobulins in juvenile rheumatoid arthritis. *Arthritis and Rheumatism.* 20:729, 1977.

noted was that girls with JRA had a higher incidence of ANA than did boys.[17,18] A larger study confirmed this and extended the correlations directly to younger age of onset and presence of iridocyclitis, and inversely to systemic disease.[19] Schaller et al.[20] have strongly emphasized the association with iridocyclitis. This appears to be most important in girls with early age of onset and pauciarticular disease, who may have as high as a 95% incidence of iridocyclitis when the ANA titer is 1/20 or greater (see Chapters 11 and 12).[21]

The nonspecific nature of the tests for ANA reduces diagnostic usefulness despite these clinical correlations. Many patients with ANA do not develop eye disease and a few with ANA do have systemic disease. The reasons are simply that nuclei are complex chemical structures with multiple potential antigens. Several isolated and reasonably pure nuclear materials have been found to be strong antigens for antibodies which characterize specific diseases or syndromes: DNA-histone, the LE cell phenomenon; native DNA, the nephritis of SLE; RNP (ribonucleoprotein), the mixed connective tissue disease; Sm (a nonhistone protein), SLE.

Despite the importance of a better understanding of pathogenesis and of increased diagnostic precision no one nuclear material has yet been found to be associated with JRA in general, with any of the subgroups, or with iridocyclitis. Attempts have been made. Before the association of ANA and iridocyclitis in JRA was recognized, Epstein et al. had reported an association with antibody to RNA and uveitis (including iridocyclitis) in a variety of contexts.[22] Using different assays Schaller et al.[20] and Schur et al.[23] found some patients with JRA had anti-RNA antibodies, but no correlations with iridocyclitis were found. Anti-DNA antibodies were found in a small proportion of children with JRA by Schaller et al. and by Bell, Talal, and Schur,[24] but with no correlation to specific clinical states.

In a series of patients from Stanford, Alspaugh and I found small proportions (less than 5%) of patients with anti-RNP, anti-native DNA,[25] anti–single-stranded DNA, and anti-RNA in patients with JRA, but again could find no correlation with clinical features of the disease.[25] A slightly larger group (8%) had rheumatoid arthritis precipitin (RAP), an antibody to an antigen present in the nuclei and cytoplasm of a cultured line of human B lymphocytes (Wil$_2$).[26] These antibodies are characteristic of LF-positive adult rheumatoid arthritis. In children they were found in girls with relatively late age of onset, as is LF positivity, but only two of six of the RAP-positive patients were also LF-positive. None of the nine defined nuclear antigens studied was found to have an association with iridocyclitis (Table 1).

Table 1
Frequency of Specific ANA in JRA

Antibody	No. positive/ No. tested	% (+) of sera screened for ANA
Anti-Sm	0/35	0
Anti-RNP	2/35	3
Anti–SS-A	0/76	0
Anti–SS-B	0/76	0
Rheumatoid arthritis precipitin (RAP)	6/76	8
Anti–DS-DNA	3/35	5
Anti–SS-DNA	2/35	3
Anti-RNA (yeast)	1/41	2
Anti-Core RNA	1/10	2

Data from Alspaugh and Miller when 77 children were screened for ANA.[25] Usually only the 37 ANA-positive sera were tested further. Values for percentage positive given in right column are based on total number screened since these antibodies are not found in ANA-negative sera.

ANTIGEN-ANTIBODY COMPLEXES

The inability of all efforts to date to define an antigen characteristic of JRA or its subgroups obviously raises doubts about comparison with the more clearly defined antigen-antibody complex diseases of adults. It is therefore reasonable to look for evidence of immune complexes per se, but relatively few attempts have been made. A major problem exists since no single assay for complexes has been uniformly successful, much less standardized. There is some evidence that individual assays have different sensitivities for the complexes of different diseases.

Pachman has had the greatest experience. Her method measures complement consumption by sera from children with JRA.[27,28] A known amount of complement is added to heat-inactivated serum from a patient and any decrease in the amount of functional complement is assumed to be a measure of complement-fixing antigen-antibody complexes in the test serum. She has found that approximately 50% of sera from patients with JRA have complement-consuming activity and that complement consumption usually correlated with increasing disease activity.

An increase in the binding of the first component of complement (C1q) by sera from some patients with systemic and polyarticular JRA has been reported in an abstract just as this is written.[29] The most intriguing point in this work was an inverse relationship between ANA and C1q-binding activity. A direct relationship would have been expected if antinuclear antibodies were forming pathogenic complexes in the circulation.

There is no a priori reason why antigen-antibody complexes need be expected in the circulation. They could either be forming *de novo* in the inflamed joints or be so rapidly removed from the circulation at sites of inflammation that serum concentrations remain below detectable levels. Bianco et al. presented data supporting these possibilities by showing that while serum levels of functional complement activity (CH-50) were elevated in patients with JRA they and the concentrations of the individual components C3 and C4 were decreased in synovial fluid from inflamed joints.[7]

I have given 13 sera from patients with active JRA to Dr. A.N. Theofilopoulos to test for circulating complexes by the Raji cell technique.[30] One was definitely positive, (from a girl who was both LF- and ANA-positive) and two had levels just above the normal range. Studies in my laboratory with Arroyave's method for detection of the activation products of C3, C3c, and C3d, indicate that a small proportion of children with JRA have this evidence for the presence of antigen-antibody complexes.[31] In theory this method could detect complexes present only in synovial fluid or tissues while other methods depend on their presence in circulating blood.

Thus it currently appears that some children with JRA have circulating antigen-antibody complexes. Localized complexes may be present in some or all. The reported inverse relationship between ANA and the C1q binding assay for complexes raises the possibility that those children who do have evidence of antigen-antibody complexes are also those who have IgM, IgG, or IgA antiglobulins.[29] However, this relationship is speculative at this time.

T CELLS

The inconstancy of results of assays for autoantibodies and antigen-antibody complexes in JRA raises the possibility that delayed hypersensitivity mediated by T lymphocytes is responsible for at least part of the inflammation. There is no direct evidence for a role for T cells in JRA but some strong arguments can be presented.

In most rheumatic diseases there are probably abnormalities of both T cell and B cell (plasma cell precursor) functions. One system may be more important in some respects in one disease than another but the more recent interest in T cell function has led to some evidence that delayed hypersensitivity has a role in even LF-positive adult RA.

Patients with severe adult RA have had their thoracic ducts cannulated for drainage and depletion of lymphocytes, most, but not all of which are T cells.[32] The protein-containing lymph is returned to the patients after removal of the cells. Arthritis and systemic features such as rheumatoid nodules improve; reinfusion of the lymphocytes causes return of arthritis. Thus depletion of the T cells presumably causes the improvement. However, the same result can occur in SLE, more certainly a disease caused by immune complexes. Several mechanisms may be involved, i.e., concomitant removal of B cells or precipitation and loss of antigen-antibody complexes during the collection and processing of the lymph. One child has been reported to have been treated this way with no effect but the clinical description suggested that ankylosing spondylitis was as likely a diagnosis as JRA.[33]

More direct support for the role of T cells in childhood arthritis is the fact that babies or young children with no detectable immunoglobulin or B cells develop a polyarticular arthritis clinically similar to JRA.[34] It is relatively easy to postulate a mechanism involving stimulation of T cells which could produce inflammation similar to that resulting from antigen-antibody complexes.[35] T cells stimulated by antigens produce biologically active materials called lymphokines which are reasonably well characterized. These could have the following roles: *chemotactic factors* attract monocytes and neutrophils;[36] *migration inhibition factor* (MIF) prevents these cells from leaving the site of inflammation;[37] *blastogenic factor* increases the local cell population;[38] *macrophage activation factors* cause release of lysosomal enzymes;[35] inflammation-promoting prostaglandin production is stimulated;[39] synovial cells start producing collagenase, which can destroy cartilage;[40] and *osteoclast activating factor* starts to destroy bone.[41] (See Chapter 6 for details of the role of the complement system and of prostaglandins.) Although most of the activities of lymphokines have only been demonstrated in vitro injections into joints of lymphokines obtained from antigen-stimulated lymphocyte cultures in test tubes have produced arthritis in rabbits,[42] and *MIF* and *blastogenic factor* have been found in synovial fluid from adults with RA.[37] However, to my knowledge none of these materials or events has been studied or demonstrated in children.

The direct studies of T cell function which have been done in children are intriguing but difficult to interpret. Two groups have reported decreased skin reactivity in delayed hypersensitivity reactions but normal tests for the in vitro reactions which are usually considered to be equivalent.[43,44] The decrease in skin reactivity was correlated to length and severity of disease and may have been due to therapy. Jennings reported very briefly a study of 17 patients with JRA, most of them with polyarticular disease, who appeared to consist of two groups in respect to T cell numbers and function.[45] The number of T cells was estimated by the percent of peripheral blood lymphocytes which bound sheep erythrocytes to their surface, E rosettes. Ten of his patients had normal percentages of E rosettes but seven had distinctly decreased percentages. Of these seven, three had markedly depressed responses in vitro to stimulation by *phytohemagglutinin* (PHA), and one had a normal blastogenic response but poor PHA-induced cytotoxicity for chicken erythrocytes. These T cell functions had been found to be normal in the earlier studies.[43,44] Brenner, Scheinberg, and Cathcart studied six patients who had had onset of JRA as children but who included four adults, one of whom was 64 years old.[46] They also found a decreased proportion of circulating E rosettes compared to normals. The decrease was due to an increase in null cells, lymphocytes with neither T nor B cell markers. The difference was in both peripheral blood and synovial fluid. A similar change was seen in SLE. Strelkauskas, Schauf, and Dray reported similar changes in nine patients with JRA using E rosettes and a method utilizing an antihuman T cell antiserum.[47] In addition they felt there was an inverse relationship between reduced proportions of T cells and disease activity. However, the data these workers presented are a bit ambiguous because of the relatively small numbers studied and because they could be interpreted as showing an increase in absolute numbers of B cells with disease activity with but little change in real numbers of T cells.

The most significant data of this type come from Norway. Abrahamsen et al. eluted lymphocytes directly from diseased synovial tissue of 11 children with JRA who had no rheumatoid factor or ANA.[48] E rosette-forming cells were present in approximately the same proportion as in peripheral blood, 70%. Cells with surface immunoglobulin (B cells) or bearing receptors for the Fc fragment of immunoglobulin (B cells and a small percentage of T cells) were present in slightly reduced proportions, and null cells, in slightly increased proportions. The responses of the eluted lymphocytes to PHA and other nonspecific mitogens were normal. However, the authors point out that the reduction in number of B cells could be due to a more rapid than usual maturation of synovial B cells to mature plasma cells.

The study of cells in diseased synovial tissue is an advance over studies limited to peripheral blood. However, it has limitations because the cell kinetics and stage of disease in a joint are hard to define and the pathology of the synovium in children with active JRA is highly variable (Figure 3). No studies of the changes of synovial pathology with time in children are yet available. T and B cell proportions and total numbers will undoubtedly be found to change with time and progression in individual joints and with different courses of disease.

The function of T and B cells is not so easily measured. A reasonable current hypothesis suggests that suppressor T cells are decreased in autoimmune diseases. In the absence of these normal inhibitory cells, autoantibodies or auto-aggressive T lymphocytes proliferate to cause disease. Studies of suppressor lymphocyte activity in humans are just starting, and no data yet exist in regard to JRA.

An attractive animal model of arthritis holds promise of sorting out the rcles of antigen-antibody complexes versus T cells in rheumatoid arthritis of children and adults. In this model mice are systemically

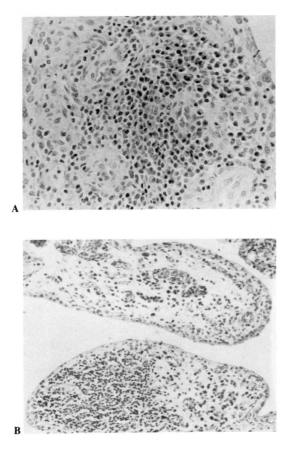

Figure 3. Photomicrographs of synovial tissue from joints of 4 children with JRA. All had exuberant synovitis resistant to drug therapy and all met criteria for synovectomy given in Chapter 16. Otherwise samples shown are unselected for type of JRA. **A.** Section of a villus showing a nodular collection of pure plasma cells. Such cells would not be typable as T or B cells but are presumably producing globulins. **B.** Sections of 2 adjacent

(*Continued*)

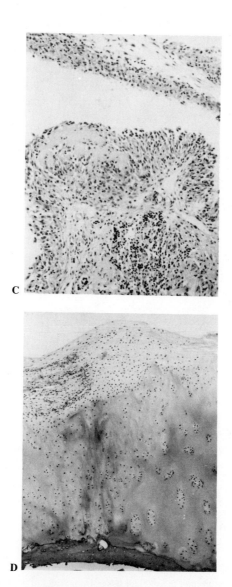

villi, one with dense infiltrate of lymphocytes and one with sparse infiltrate of plasma cells. **C.** Section of villus which, in contrast to those in Figures 3A or 3B, has marked synovial cell hyperplasia. A fibrin inclusion is seen within the piled up synovial cells. **D.** Section of cartilage at the margin of a joint which is being eroded by pannus which is relatively acellular. There is no obvious synovial cell hyperplasia.

immunized to methylated bovine serum albumin and develop chronic arthritis when this antigen is subsequently reinjected into joints. Susceptibility is genetically determined, as is probably true for RA and JRA (see Chapter 8).[49] Serum of sensitized mice can transfer susceptibility, but not as well as it does T cells.[50] In this system the arthritis is apparently T cell-dependent although ultimate expression might involve antibody production in the synovium. Even a small amount of antibody might have significant effect because of the phenomenon of antibody-dependent cellular cytotoxicity (ADCC).[35] In this in vitro process T or B cells can cause lysis of target cells in the presence of minute amounts of specific anti-target antibody. ADCC is a model of ways in which pathogenic events may be mediated by both T and B cells. It is becoming progressively attractive as a mechanism in rheumatic disease as we learn more of the involvement and interdependence of both immune systems.

SUMMARY AND SPECULATIONS

The currently recognized immunologic abnormalities in JRA are inconstant. Some children have classical IgM rheumatoid factor and a few more have increased concentrations of IgG or IgA antiglobulins without IgM rheumatoid factor. Antinuclear antibodies of unknown specificity are found independently in others. Some children evidence the presence of circulating antigen-antibody complexes, but the results of different assays vary. There are rough but imperfect correlations between presence of IgM rheumatoid factor or antinuclear antibodies and the clinical picture and prognosis. Abnormalities of T cell function are likely to be involved in all forms of JRA. Studies to date suggest these patients develop a state of decreased skin reactivity but have and maintain normal in vitro correlations of delayed hypersensitivity. These studies have not yet been very helpful diagnostically or in regard to understanding pathogenesis.

Until recently discussions of the classifications of types of JRA have been dependent almost exclusively on clinical presentation but it would be far more satisfactory if we could establish diagnostic groups and subgroups by laboratory data. The available tests are helpful: LF to determine prognosis for bad joint disease and ANA to predict a risk for iridocyclitis. However, all available laboratory data lack definition: we do not know the prognostic implications of IgG antiglobulins in the absence of IgM rheumatoid factor in children or whether a specific antibody is involved in iridocyclitis. Eventually the presence of specific immunologic abnormalities may provide a more rational and precise way to categorize the diseases now grouped as JRA.

48

REFERENCES

1. Bywaters, E.G.L., Carter, M.E., and Scott, F.E.T. Differential agglutination titre (DAT) in juvenile rheumatoid arthritis. *Ann Rheum Dis.* 18:225–38, 1959.

2. Laaksonen, A.-L. A prognostic study of juvenile rheumatoid arthritis. *Acta Paediatr Scand.* 116 (suppl):38–41, 1966.

3. Cassidy, J.T., and Valkenburg, H.A. A five year prospective study of rheumatoid factor tests in juvenile rheumatoid arthritis. *Arthritis Rheum.* 10:83–90, 1967.

4. Hanson, V., Drexler, E., and Kornreich, H. The relationship of rheumatoid factor to age of onset in juvenile rheumatoid arthritis. *Arthritis Rheum.* 12:82–6, 1969.

5. Torrigiani, G., Ansell, B.M., Chown, E.E.A., and Roitt, I.M. Raised IgG antiglobulin factors in Still's disease. *Ann Rheum Dis.* 28:424–7, 1969.

6. Florin-Christensen, A., Arana, R.M., Morteo, O.G. et al. IgG, IgA, IgM and IgD antiglobulins in juvenile rheumatoid arthritis. *Ann Rheum Dis.* 33:32–4, 1974.

7. Bianco, N.E., Panush, R.S., Stillman, J.S., and Schur, P.H. Immunologic studies of juvenile rheumatoid arthritis. *Arthritis Rheum.* 14:685–96, 1971.

8. Bianco, N.E., Dobkin, L.W., and Schur, P.H. Immunological properties of isolated IgG and IgM anti-gammaglobulins (rheumatoid factors). *Clin Exp Immunol.* 17:91–101, 1974.

9. Munthe, E. Anti-IgG and antinuclear antibodies in juvenile rheumatoid arthritis. *Scand J Rheumatol.* 1:161–70, 1972.

10. Munthe, E. Complexes of IgG and IgG rheumatoid factor in synovial tissues of juvenile rheumatoid arthritis. *Scand J Rheumatol.* 1:153–60, 1972.

11. Miller, J.J. III, Olds-Arroyo, L., and Akasaka, T. Antiglobulins in juvenile rheumatoid arthritis. *Arthritis Rheum.* 20:729–35, 1977.

12. Moore, T., Dorner, R.W., and Zuckner, J. Hidden rheumatoid factors in seronegative juvenile rheumatoid arthritis. *Ann Rheum Dis.* 33:255–7, 1974.

13. Beck, J.S. Auto-antibodies to cell nuclei. *Scott Med J.* 10:373–88, 1963.

14. Hasker, J., Mackay, I.R., and Miller, J.J. III. The incidence of "antinuclear factor" in human disease. *Australas Ann Med.* 14:96–101, 1965.

15. Barnett, E.V., North, A.F., Jr., Condemi, J.C. et al. Antinuclear factors in systemic lupus erythematosus and rheumatoid arthritis. *Ann Intern Med.* 63:100–8, 1965.

16. Rosenberg, J.N., Johnson, G.D., Holborow, E.J., and Bywaters, E.G.L. Eosinophil-specific and other granulocyte-specific antinuclear antibodies in juvenile chronic polyarthritis and adult rheumatoid arthritis. *Ann Rheum Dis.* 34:350–53, 1975.

17. Miller, J.J. III, Henrich, V.L., and Brandstrup, N.E. Sex difference in incidence of antinuclear factors in juvenile rheumatoid arthritis. *Pediatrics.* 38:916–18, 1966.

18. Kornreich, H.K., Drexler, E., and Hanson, V. Antinuclear factors in childhood rheumatic diseases. *J Pediatr.* 69:1039–45, 1966.

19. Petty, R.E., Cassidy, J.T., and Sullivan, D.B. Clinical correlates of

antinuclear antibodies in juvenile rheumatoid arthritis. *J Pediatr.* 83:386–89, 1973.

20. Schaller, J.G., Johnson, G.D., Holborow, E.J. et al. The association of antinuclear antibodies with the chronic iridocyclitis of juvenile rheumatoid arthritis (Still's Disease). *Arthritis Rheum.* 17:409–16, 1974.

21. Chylack, L.T., Jr. The ocular manifestations of juvenile rheumatoid arthritis. *Arthritis Rheum.* 20 (suppl):217–23, 1977.

22. Epstein, W.V., Tan, M., and Easterbrook, M. Serum antibody to double-stranded RNA and DNA in patients with idiopathic and secondary uveitis. *N Engl J Med.* 285:1502–6, 1971.

23. Schur, P.H., Stollar, B.D., Steinberg, A.D., and Talal, N. Incidence of antibody to double-stranded RNA in systemic lupus erythematosus and related diseases. *Arthritis Rheum.* 14:342–7, 1971.

24. Bell, C., Talal, N., and Schur, P.H. Antibodies to DNA in patients with rheumatoid arthritis and juvenile rheumatoid arthritis. *Arthritis Rheum.* 18:535–40, 1975.

25. Alspaugh, M.A., and Miller, J.J. III. A study of specificities of antinuclear antibodies in juvenile rheumatoid arthritis. *J Pediatr.* 90:391–5, 1977.

26. Alspaugh, M.A., and Tan, E.M. Serum antibody in rheumatoid arthritis reactive with a cell-associated antigen. *Arthritis Rheum.* 19:711–19, 1976.

27. Pachman, L.M., Baldwin, S.M., and Gaekwar, S.M. Anticomplementary activity of sera from patients with juvenile rheumatoid arthritis, rheumatoid arthritis, systemic lupus erythematosus, and normal controls, abstracted. *Pediatr Res.* 9:333, 1975.

28. Pachman, L.M., and Baldwin, S.M. Assays of complement in polyarticular juvenile rheumatoid arthritis. *Arthritis Rheum.* 20 (suppl):467–70, 1977.

29. Person, D.A., Brewer, E.J., and Rossen, R.D. Immune complexes and antinuclear antibodies in sera from patients with juvenile rheumatoid arthritis, abstracted. *Clin Res.* 25:365A, 1977.

30. Theofilopoulos, A.N., Wilson, C.B., and Bokisch, V.A. Binding of soluble immune complexes to human lymphoblastoid cells. II. Use of Raji cells to detect circulating immune complexes in animal and human sera. *J Exp Med.* 140:1230–44, 1974.

31. Arroyave, C.M., and Tan, E.M. Detection of complement activation by counter-immunoelectrophoresis (CIE). *J Immunol Methods.* 13:101–12, 1976.

32. Pearson, C.M., Paulus, H.E., and Machleder, H.I. The role of lymphocyte and its products in the propagation of joint disease. *Ann NY Acad Sci.* 256:150–68, 1975.

33. Wegelius, O., Laine, V., Lindstrom, B., and Klockars, M. Fistula of the thoracic duct as an immunosuppressive treatment in rheumatoid arthritis. *Acta Med Scand.* 187:539–44, 1970.

34. Good, R.A., Venters, H., Page, A.R., and Good, T.A. Diffuse connective tissue diseases in childhood. *Journal Lancet.* 81:192–204, 1961.

35. Waksman, B.H. Commentary: immunoglobulins and lymphokines as mediators of inflammatory cell mobilization and target cell killing. *Cell Immunol.* 27:309–15, 1976.

36. Ward, P.A., Remold, H.G., and David, J.R. Leukotactic factor produced by sensitized lymphocytes. *Science.* 163:1079–81, 1969.

50

37. Stastny, P., Rosenthal, M., Andreis, M., and Ziff, M. Lymphokines in the rheumatoid joint. *Arthritis Rheum.* 18:237–43, 1975.

38. Maini, R.N., Bryceson, A.D.M., and Wolstencroft, R.A. Lymphocyte mitogenic factor in man. *Nature.* 224:43–4, 1969.

39. Dayer, J.-M., Robinson, D.R., and Krane, S.M. Prostaglandin production by rheumatoid synovial cells. Stimulation by a factor from human mononuclear cells. *J Exp Med.* 145:1399–1404, 1977.

40. Dayer, J.-M., Russell, R.G.G., and Krane, S.M. Collagenase production by rheumatoid synovial cells: stimulation by a human lymphocyte factor. *Science.* 195:181–3, 1977.

41. Horton, J.E., Raisz, L.G., Simmons, H.A. et al. Bone resorbing activity in supernatant fluid from cultured human peripheral blood leukocytes. *Science.* 177:793–5, 1972.

42. Andreis, M., Stastny, P., and Ziff, M. Experimental arthritis produced by injection of mediators of delayed hypersensitivity. *Arthritis Rheum.* 17:537–51, 1974.

43. Panush, R.S., Bianco, N.E., Schur, P.H. et al. Juvenile rheumatoid arthritis: cellular hypersensitivity and selective IgA deficiency. *Clin Exp Immunol.* 10:103–15, 1972.

44. Høyeraal, H.M., Frøland, S.S., and Wisløff, F. Lymphocyte populations and cellular immune reactions in juvenile rheumatoid arthritis. *Scand J Immunol.* 4:801–10, 1975.

45. Jennings, J. Defective cellular immunity in juvenile rheumatoid arthritis. *Ann Rheum Dis.* 34:196, 1975.

46. Brenner, A.I., Scheinberg, M.A., and Cathcart, E.S. Surface characteristics of synovial fluid and peripheral blood lymphocytes in inflammatory arthritis. *Arthritis Rheum.* 18:297–303, 1975.

47. Strelkauskas, A.J., Schauf, V., and Dray, S. Alterations in T, B, and null cells in children with autoimmune diseases. *Clin Immunol Immunopathol.* 6:359–68, 1976.

48. Abrahamsen, T.G., Frøland, S.S., Natvig, J.B., and Pahle, J. Lymphocytes eluted from synovial tissue of juvenile rheumatoid arthritis patients. *Arthritis Rheum.* 20:772–8, 1977.

49. Brackertz, D., Mitchell, G.F., and Mackay, I.R. Antigen-induced arthritis in mice. I. Induction of arthritis in various strains of mice. *Arthritis Rheum.* 20:841–50, 1977.

50. Brackertz, D., Mitchell, G.F., Vadas, M.A., and Mackay, I.R. Studies on antigen-induced arthritis in mice. III. Cell and serum transfer experiments. *J Immunol.* 118:1645–8, 1977.

5 Immunodeficiency and Arthritis

Ross E. Petty

An association between immunodeficiencies and rheumatic diseases is increasingly recognized. Early observations of the occurrence of "collagen disease" in agammaglobulinemia[1,2] were followed by reports of increased frequency of immunoglobulin A deficiency,[3,4] complement deficiencies,[5] and neutrophil[6] and macrophage[7] abnormalities in a variety of inflammatory rheumatic diseases.[1-7] Recognition of more subtle quantitative and qualitative immunodeficiencies either as primary or secondary phenomena has resulted in additional associations with rheumatic diseases.

The reported associations between relatively well-defined immunodeficiencies and juvenile rheumatoid arthritis (JRA) are summarized in Table I.

HYPOGAMMAGLOBULINEMIA AND CHRONIC OLIGOARTICULAR ARTHRITIS

An association between immune deficiencies and rheumatic diseases was first noted only four years after the description of hypogammaglobulinemia by Bruton.[8] Janeway,[1,9] and others[2,3,10-12] noted in the occurrence of a chronic noninfectious inflammatory oligoarthritis in patients with congenital or acquired hypogammaglobulinemia. The actual incidence of rheumatic disease in hypogammaglobulinemia has been studied by several observers.[2,10-16] In a review of 58 reported cases of hypogammaglobulinemia up to 1957, arthritis was described in eight, a prevalence of 13.8%.[2] Some of these patients, however, had septic arthritis or arthritis apparently related to infection elsewhere which subsided with antibiotic therapy. Lawrence reported that four of 60 males with hypogammaglobulinemia had chronic inflammatory arthritis, three others had synovitis of the knees, and four had had polyarthritis in the past.[11,12]

Schaller, McLaughlin et al. found a much lower incidence with arthritis in one of eight boys with X-linked agammaglobulinemia and none of 10 children with non–X-linked hypogammaglobulinemia.[13,14] In studies of 29 patients with hypogammaglobulinemia, chronic oligoarthritis was found in three of eight boys with familial (i.e., X-linked) hypogammaglobulinemia and in three of 21 patients without a family history of immunodeficiency.[15,16] The joint disease seen in these patients was clinically indistinguishable from pauciarticular JRA. Between three and 15 years of age there was onset of arthritis in one to four large peripheral joints characterized by a moderate to large amount of synovial fluid, soft tissue thickening, and limitation of mo-

Table I
Immunodeficiency and Chronic Arthritis

Immunodeficiency	Incidence of Arthritis	Author
Hypogammaglobulinemia	6/16	Janeway et al.[1,9]
Hypogammaglobulinemia	8/27	Good et al.[10]
Hypogammaglobulinemia	4/60	Lawrence et al.[11,12]
Hypogammaglobulinemia	1/18	Schaller et al.[13,14]
Hypogammaglobulinemia	6/29	Petty et al.[15,16]
Selective IgA deficiency	14/324	Cassidy et al.[3,25,26]
Selective IgA deficiency	2/23	Huntley et al.[4]
Selective IgA deficiency	3/176	Panush et al.[30]
Selective IgA deficiency	11/300	Pelkonen et al.[32]
Nezelof's syndrome	1/3	Tubergen[37]
Wiskott-Aldrich syndrome	4/18	Cooper et al.[38]
Wiskott-Aldrich syndrome	2/4	Schaller et al.[14]
Immunodeficiency with thymoma	1	Adler[39]
C2 deficiency	10/274	Glass et al.[40]

Superscripts indicate references.

tion. Pain and stiffness were frequently mild. Laboratory studies of such individuals revealed that none had rheumatoid factors, antinuclear antibody, bony erosions, or rheumatoid nodules. Synovial fluid contained a moderate number of mononuclear cells and microscopy of the synovium showed moderate hyperplasia, hypertrophy, vascular endothelial proliferation, and subsynovial proliferation of fibrous tissue, but without marked infiltration by lymphocytes or plasma cells.[1,15,18]

In addition to chronic oligoarthritis, most reports indicate transient recurrent arthralgia or arthritis in patients with either congenital or acquired hypogammaglobulinemia.[8,11,14,15] In fact, the original patient described by Bruton presented with pain in the knee.[8] Although both clinically and on the basis of synovial fluid analysis and synovial membrane histology arthritis associated with hypogammaglobulinemia is highly similar to JRA, it should not be assumed that they are identical diseases. For example, the strong association between pauciarticular JRA and uveitis has not been reported in the pauciarticular arthritis of hypogammaglobulinemia.[19,20] The low incidence of rheumatoid nodules and erosive arthritis in hypogammaglobulinemic patients with arthritis is not in itself surprising, however, since in comparable pauciarticular JRA without hypogammaglobulinemia such abnormalities are unusual.[19,21]

Management of arthritis of the hypogammaglobulinemic patient is no different from that of JRA. The arthritis of some patients apparently responds to replacement of gamma globulin[17] but in other instances, it persists in spite of intensive treatment with intramuscular Cohn fraction II, plasma, or intravenous plasmin-treated Cohn fraction II.[15,16] In one series, in five of the six hypogammaglobulinemic patients with arthritis, joint disease began months to years after gamma globulin replacement therapy for recurrent infection began.[15,16] These discrepancies probably represent heterogeneity of the arthritides associated with hypogammaglobulinemia. It may also result from the fact that in many patients hypogammaglobulinemia is not the only immunodeficiency, there being significant evidence of impaired thymus-dependent lymphocyte function and neutropenia in many.[15,16,22] These abnormalities may play a role in pathogenesis of arthritis and are largely unaffected by gamma globulin replacement.

IMMUNOGLOBULIN-A DEFICIENCY AND RHEUMATIC DISEASES

The prevalence of immunoglobulin-A (IgA) deficiency, the most common immunodeficiency in man, depends upon definition. When patients with serum IgA less than 0.01 mg/ml are designated IgA-deficient, the incidence varies from 0.097% in a large community survey[23] to 0.250% in blood donors.[24] (The associations between IgA deficiency and JRA and other rheumatic diseases are summarized in Table I.)

In one study 14 of 324 patients with JRA had serum IgA less than 0.01 mg/ml and undetectable secretory IgA, but normal or increased levels of IgG and IgM.[26] A similar incidence has been demonstrated in systemic lupus erythematosus (SLE) and rheumatoid arthritis;[27] and individuals with IgA deficiency and dermatomyositis, Raynaud's phenomenon, and ankylosing spondylitis have been reported,[28,29] although no exact incidence data are available. It appears, therefore, that the incidence of IgA deficiency in rheumatic diseases including JRA is approximately 40 times higher than in community survey populations and 20 times that present in blood donors, although there may be regional differences in their incidence. In addition, there is an increased incidence of low, but detectable levels of IgA in patients with JRA.[26]

As in patients with hypogammaglobulinemia, arthritis in patients with IgA deficiency is clinically indistinguishable from JRA in non–IgA-deficient patients. In contrast to arthritis associated with hypogammaglobulinemia, that found in IgA-deficient patients may be pauciarticular or polyarticular, and iridocyclitis is not infrequent. Furthermore, antinuclear antibodies and rheumatoid factor may be present.[25,26] In one instance administration of plasma to an IgA-deficient patient with chronic deforming erosive arthritis affecting small and large peripheral joints, temporomandibular joints, and cervical spine, was followed by decrease in activity of the joint disease.[31] Eleven months after the last plasma infusion, the patient had, for the first time, detectable IgA in secretions and low normal IgA levels in serum. Whether or not infusion of plasma directly affected the course of this patient's disease or the establishment of endogenous IgA production is not known. With rare exceptions IgA deficiency is thought to be congenital and permanent, although proof that the IgA-deficient patient never had serum or secretory IgA is usually lacking.[32]

Two aspects of IgA deficiency are especially relevant to rheumatic diseases and merit further comment: the occurrence of anti-IgA antibodies, and of antibodies to native DNA. Hemagglutinating anti-IgA antibodies were found in one-third of IgA-deficient individuals with nonrheumatic diseases, in three-quarters of IgA deficient patients with JRA, and in all of the IgA-deficient patients with SLE.[29] Such antibodies to IgA were not demonstrated in patients with rheumatic diseases and normal or increased levels of IgA, in patients with hypogammaglobulinemia, or in normal individuals.[29] Thus IgA-deficient patients with rheumatic diseases may be at increased risk to develop anti-IgA antibodies. Such antibodies have been implicated in transfusion reactions, and IgA-deficient blood product recipients with rheumatic diseases may therefore be at risk from blood products containing IgA.[33]

Antinuclear antibodies (ANA) occurred in 71% of one group of IgA-deficient patients with JRA.[26] Although this is considerably higher when compared to reported incidences in groups of patients with JRA it is probably related to the fewer numbers of patients with systemic onset of disease (where ANA is uncommon) and to the relatively high incidence of uveitis where ANA is common.[19,20]

It has been asserted that as a group, patients with IgA deficiency have a high incidence of antibody to native DNA.[34] Patients in whom this observation was made were asymptomatic and thought not to have SLE. Other reports have failed to confirm this observation.[35,36]

THYMUS-DEPENDENT IMMUNODEFICIENCIES AND ARTHRITIS

Although the commonest immunodeficiencies found in association with rheumatic diseases are hypogammaglobulinemia and IgA deficiency, note should be made of several others. One patient with Nezelof's syndrome, (lymphopenic immunodeficiency with normal immunoglobulins) had autoimmune thyroiditis, autoimmune hemolytic anemia, thrombocytopenia, and severe JRA affecting many joints including temporomandibular joints and cervical spine. Neither of two affected siblings had joint disease. Administration of transfer factor and fetal thymus transplantation failed to affect the joint disease or permanently reconstitute T lymphocyte function.[37]

Arthritis has been reported in association with Wiskott-Aldrich syndrome, another immunodeficiency syndrome with T lymphocyte impairment. Four of 18 patients reviewed by Cooper et al.[38] had transient or recurrent arthritis, two of four patients followed by Schaller[14] had similar disease, and a single patient with the rare syndrome of immunodeficiency with thymoma was reported to have arthritis.[39]

COMPLEMENT DEFICIENCIES AND ARTHRITIS

Primary deficiencies of complement components are associated with rheumatic diseases. Deficiencies of C1r, C1s, C2, C4, C5 and C1 INH have all been associated with SLE (reviewed by Schur[41]), but the most common complement component deficiency associated with JRA is

58

of antinuclear antibodies with chronic iridocyclitis of juvenile rheumatoid arthritis (Still's disease). *Arthritis Rheum.* 17:409–16, 1974.

21. Hanson, V., Drexler, E., and Kornreich, H. The relationship of rheumatoid factor to age of onset of juvenile rheumatoid arthritis. *Arthritis Rheum.* 12:86–7, 1969.

22. Rosen, F.S. Immunological Deficiency Disease. Edited by F.H. Bach, and R.A. Good. In *Clinical Immunology.* New York: Academic Press, 1972, p. 271.

23. Cassidy, J.T., and Nordby, G.L. Human serum immunoglobulin concentrations: prevalence of immunoglobulin deficiencies. *J Allergy Clin Immunol.* 55:35–48, 1975.

24. Koistinen, J. Selective IgA deficiency in blood donors. *Vox Sang.* 29:192–202, 1975.

25. Cassidy, J.T., Petty, R.E., and Sullivan, D.B. Abnormalities in the distribution of serum immunoglobulin concentrations in juvenile rheumatoid arthritis. *J Clin Invest.* 52:1931–6, 1973.

26. Cassidy, J.T., Petty, R.E., and Sullivan, D.B. The occurrence of selective IgA deficiency in children with juvenile rheumatoid arthritis. *Arthritis Rheum.* 20 (suppl):181–3, 1977.

27. Cassidy, J.T., Burt, A., Petty, R.E., and Sullivan, D.B. Prevalence of selective IgA deficiency in patients with connective tissue disease. *N Engl J Med.* 280:275, 1969.

28. Ammann, A.J., and Hong, R. Selective IgA deficiency: presentation of 30 cases and a review of the literature. *Medicine.* 50:223–36, 1971.

29. Petty, R.E., Palmer, N.R., Cassidy, J.T. et al. The association of autoimmune diseases and anti-IgA antibodies in patients with selective IgA deficiency. *Clin. Res.* 24:543A, 1976.

30. Panush, R.S., Bianco, N.E., Schur, P.H. et al. Juvenile rheumatoid arthritis, cellular hypersensitivity and selective IgA deficiency. *Clin Exp Immunol.* 10:103–15, 1972.

31. Petty, R.E., Cassidy, J.T., and Sullivan, D.B. Reversal of selective IgA deficiency in a child with juvenile rheumatoid arthritis after plasma transfusions. *Pediatrics.* 51:44–8, 1973.

32. Pelkonen, P., Savilahti, E., Westeren, L., and Makela, A.L. IgA deficiency in juvenile rheumatoid arthritis. *Scand J Rheumatol.* 8 (suppl): 4–13, 1975.

33. Leikola, J., Koistinen, J., Lehtinen, M., and Virolainen, M. IgA-induced anaphylactic transfusion reactions: a report of four cases. *Blood.* 42:111–19, 1973.

34. Gershwin, M.E., Blaese, R.M., Steinberg, A.D. et al. Antibodies to nucleic acids in congenital immune deficiencies. *J Pediatr.* 89:377–81, 1976.

35. Petty, R.E., Cassidy, J.T., and Tubergen, D.G. The disease association of antibody to double-stranded DNA in patients with selective IgA deficiency. *Clin Res.* 24:543A, 1976.

36. Amman, A.J., Wara, D.W., Pillarisetty, R.J., and Talal, N. Autoantibody, autoimmune disease and immunodeficiency. *Arthritis Rheum.* 20 (suppl):438–40, 1977.

37. Tubergen, D.G. Thymus transplant in lymphopenic immune deficiency (Nezelof's syndrome). *J Pediatr.* 84:915, 1974.

38. Cooper, M.D., Chase, H.P., Lowman, J.T. et al. Wiskott-Aldrich syndrome: an immunologic deficiency disease involving the afferent limb of immunity. *Am J Med.* 44:499–513, 1968.

39. Adler, E., and Gehrmann, G. Blutkrankheiten nach thymus–tumor-extirpation. *Dtsch Med Wochenschr*. 92:423, 1967.

40. Glass, D., Raum, D., Gibson, D. et al. Inherited deficiency of the second component of complement: rheumatic disease associations. *J Clin Invest*. 58:853–61, 1976.

41. Schur, P.H. Complement in lupus. *Clin Rheum Dis*. 1:519–43, 1975.

42. Osofsky, S.G., Thompson, B.H., Lint, T.F., and Gewurz, H. Hereditary deficiency of the third component of complement in a child with fever, skin rash and arthralgias. Response to transfusions of whole blood. *J Pediatr*. 90:180–6, 1977.

43. Howie, J.B., and Helyer, B.J. The immunology and pathology of NZB mice. *Adv Immunol*. 9:215–66, 1968.

44. Oldstone, M.B.A., and Dixon, F.J. Pathogenesis of chronic disease associated with persistent lymphocytic choriomeningitis viral infection. *J Exp Med*. 131:1–14, 1970.

45. Soothill, J.F., and Steward, M.W. The immunopathological significance of the heterogeneity of antibody affinity. *Clin Exp Immunol*. 9:193–9, 1970.

46. Petty, R.E., and Steward, M.W. Relative affinity of anti-protein antibodies in New Zealand mice. *Clin Exp Immunol*. 12:343–50, 1972.

47. Petty, R.E., and Steward, M.W. The relationship of antibody affinity to onset of immune-complex disease in New Zealand mice. *Ann Rheum Dis*. 36:39–43, 1977.

48. Scheinberg, M.A., Mendes, N.F., Kopersztych, S., and Cathcart, E.S. Clinical applications of T, B and K cell determinations in rheumatic diseases: a review. *Semin Arthritis Rheum*. 6:1–18, 1976.

49. Kass, E., Frøland, S.S., Natvig, J.B. et al. Transfer factor in juvenile rheumatoid arthritis. *Lancet* 1:627, 1974.

50. Schuermans, Y. Levamisole in rheumatoid arthritis. *Lancet* 1:111, 1975.

6 Complement and Soluble Mediators of Inflammation in JRA

Lauren M. Pachman

Many soluble mediators of inflammation have been characterized in recent years, encompassing both humoral and cellular products. In this chapter specific evidence derived from patients with JRA concerning the interaction of immune complexes with both the complement system and the phagocyte will be reviewed. The role of two other major contributors to inflammation will be considered: the clotting system and prostaglandins. Recent evidence from adult rheumatologic studies suggests that additional investigation in these areas will be needed to obtain data about soluble mediators of inflammation in JRA.

Interpretation of the available data concerning JRA may be confounded by several factors: (1) the age of onset of the disease may have been in childhood but the reported testing performed in the afflicted adult; (2) there may be no mention of disease activity or relationship of therapy to the time of testing; and (3) the group defined as JRA is a heterogeneous one. For example, the syndromes of seronegative spondylitis include psoriasis, ulcerative colitis, Crohn's disease, and Reiter's disease, thus indicating the heterogeneity of rheumatoid factor-negative disease that involves the back.[1] Recent evidence has been presented that HLA-B27–positive patients with ankylosing spondylitis do not have circulating immune complexes which either bind to C1q or cause increased breakdown products of C3.[2] It is now recognized that a subgroup of patients with JRA have this disease. Therefore, it is possible that *all* subgroups of rheumatoid arthritis in children may not be classified as immune complex disease. Nevertheless, it remains a working hypothesis with which to organize the current concepts of pathogenesis.

THE ROLE OF COMPLEMENT IN JRA

A leading theory is that JRA is an immune complex disease in which a large component of tissue damage is achieved via activation of complement and augmented by cellular enzyme release. The main basis of this theory stems from the observation that hemolytic complement levels (CH50) in synovial fluid may be decreased in children with rheumatoid factor-negative disease, similar to those found in rheumatoid factor-positive fluid.[3-7]

It is well established that complexes of IgG-IgG or IgG-IgM bind to the first component of complement directly, activating the classical complement cascade and generating complement fragments which then interact with a variety of cellular and humoral elements. The structure and function of the components of the complement system has recently been reviewed and is an area of intensive investigation by several laboratories.[8] Inasmuch as 80% of sera from children with JRA do not have IgM rheumatoid factor by conventional testing, it is pertinent to examine the evidence that complexes of IgG-IgG activate the complement system in clinical disease.

Evidence that IgG Complexes Activate Complement

The finding that IgG and C3 are deposited in rheumatoid synovium of affected joints in children,[9] as they are in adults,[10-12] and are associated with intraarticular depletion of complement, supports the belief that immune complexes containing IgG activate the complement system.[9,13] The capacity to activate complement is thought to be due in part to aggregate size as well as to the specific composition of the complex. Aggregated tightly bound IgG was detected in some fluids with low total hemolytic complement and was not correlated with serum level of IgM rheumatoid factor.[14] The final size of the aggregate produced may be a function of the tendency of specific IgG molecules to selfassociation,[15] as well as of the binding to IgG producing plasma cells in the synovium of IgG present in the fluid phase, binding intracellular C1q and C3.[16] The decrease in complement components in the synovial fluid varied directly with the amount of IgG complexes present. The quantity of the 7S gammaglobulin complexes was inversely related to the CH50, and C1q or C3 P-A levels. Furthermore, fluid with abundant complexes manifested an anticomplementary activity which was enhanced by 7S rheumatoid factor indicating that IgG was present, and formed a distinct precipitate when isolated C1q was added to the individual synovial fluid, documenting its ability to bind to the first component of complement.[17]

Synovial Fluid Complement Levels in JRA

Bianco, et al. found in a study of 148 patients with the diagnosis of JRA that synovial fluid from three of 15 rheumatoid factor-positive patients had lower levels of C3 and C4 as well as CH50.[5] Synovial fluids from 13 patients with rheumatoid negative fluid were studied but it was not stated if levels of complement were decreased relative to normal controls. These authors did find increased amounts of IgA and IgG antiglobulins in children with JRA. Those who had rheumatoid factor-negative joint fluid usually had elevated levels of serum complement and an acute pauciarticular, self-limited course.

Ruddy assayed paired serum and synovial fluid specimens from 18 children (8 females and 10 males) with a clinical diagnosis of JRA and measured the CH50, C1, C4, C2 and C9, and total protein content.[6] The levels of C4 proved to be the most sensitive index of complement activation. The patients were divided into two groups, depending on the synovial fluid titer of C4. Group I had low synovial levels of C4, tended to be females with polyarticular disease, and of older age at onset; only three of the eight were rheumatoid factor-positive. However, serum C4 was not depressed, suggesting intraarticular complement consumption. The second group had normal synovial fluid levels of C4, consisted of more males than females, who in general had pauciarticular disease. No significant differences were found in either the levels of C1 or C2 activity in synovial fluid or sera from either of the two groups. The level of C9 was usually elevated to twice that observed in normal controls and was correlated with the erythrocyte sedimentation rate.[6]

Similar evidence of complement activation is derived from studies of synovial fluid from populations which include both rheumatoid factor-negative and rheumatoid factor-positive adults, but in which the age of onset of the disease was not specified and hence may not truly reflect the juvenile rheumatoid population. Using a method which detects complexes by their ability to bind to isolated labeled C1q, Lambert et al. found that 65% of rheumatoid factor-positive patients had increased binding, and that binding was increased in 67% of rheumatoid factor-negative sera as well.[18] A significant correlation was found between ^{125}I-C1q binding capacity and synovial C4 levels. No correlation was found with levels of C3. Breakdown products of C3 and C3PA were found in 90% of both rheumatoid factor-negative and -positive synovial fluids, suggesting complement activation is similar in both forms of the disease.[18,19] However, 44% of nine samples from patients with other types of inflammatory arthritis were positive for C3 fragments, indicating the lack of specificity of this determination versus that of C1q binding which was positive only in immune complex disease and not in inflammatory arthritis.[18]

In a recent study of serum and synovial fluid obtained from 20 children with definite JRA, direct evidence has been provided indicating that intraarticular complement activation proceeds by the classical rather than alternate pathway. Using assays of specific functional activity of the complement components, Rynes, Ruddy, Spragg, et al. found that synovial fluid CH50, C1, C4 and C2 correlated significantly and CH50 had the closest correlation with levels of C1.[20] Measurement of the concentrations of properdin factors B and P, as well as kininogins were not abnormal in synovial fluid obtained from involved joints. These observations suggest that the classical pathway is the most involved in complement activation in rheumatoid factor-negative JRA.

Intraarticular complement depletion is thought to be a consequence of binding of complement by immune complexes. Only a few studies have been performed in children in which the histologic evidence of complement deposition was correlated with synovial levels of complement. In one such study intraarticular complement levels in eight children and seven adults with rheumatoid arthritis were correlated with the immunopathology of the joint.[9] Only three of the children had low synovial/serum complement ratios. This depression was not related to rheumatoid factor positivity or histologic evidence of intraarticular deposition of immunoglobulin or complement, thus leaving the question concerning the ultimate fate of complement unsettled.

It has been noted that immune deposits of IgM, complement and fibrinogen may be present in the skin as well as in the joints. When uninvolved skin from 40 patients with rheumatoid arthritis was biopsied, immune deposits localized to the dermal-epidermal junction were found which correlated positively with the presence of cryoglobulins, but complement levels were not reported and no seronegative children with JRA were studied.[20]

Complement Levels in Sera of Patients with JRA

As in adults,[22] measurements of total hemolytic complement levels in sera of children with JRA have demonstrated a higher than "normal" range in many studies.[23,24] One difficulty in interpreting the results completely has been the lack of normal complement levels in the pediatric range. Recent work has indicated that the total hemolytic complement does not vary with age but that the absolute amount of complement components of either the direct[25,26] or alternate pathway may be age-related.[27] It was suggested that change with time of a specific test may offer the most information concerning the progress of a disease in an individual child.[25]

Several pediatric studies have measured complement components in sera taken from patients with JRA. One survey showed a slight increase in C4 in active disease.[28] In another study of 100 children with JRA in which C3 was the only complement component measured, no correlation with disease activity was noted.[29] This finding was echoed by another study in which single, nonsequential observations were also obtained.[30] One investigator noted that a low serum complement was usually associated with rheumatoid factor-positive polyarticular disease, increased nodules, and prolonged course.[5] Høyeraal presented values obtained from 35 hospitalized patients with JRA which were paired with those from age and sex matched controls.[24] This study did not substantiate reports of low levels of CH50 in children with rheumatoid factor-positive arthritis.[5] Instead, significantly higher serum levels of CH50, C3, C4 and C3 P-A were measured although the amount of C1q was the same for both rheumatoid factor-positive and rheumatoid factor-negative children. It was hypothesized that increase in consumption resulted in increased complement formation with overcompensation.[24] Substantiation of this concept may be derived from other studies in which there was an inverse relationship between the total hemolytic complement of patients with JRA and the amount of complement consumption.[31] When clinical response to therapy was achieved, complement consumption fell and the total hemolytic complement rose.[32] It was observed that fluctuations of total hemolytic complement occurred within the normal range so that serial observations were often more useful laboratory correlates of clinical disease.[33]

Activation of a Complement Source by Sera of Patients with JRA

An assay which inactivates the heat-labile endogenous complement present in test sera has been used to study the amount of anticomplementary activity or complement consuming factor(s) present in the sera of patients with definite JRA. The difference between the amount of complement in the source added to the incubation mixture as opposed to that found *after* incubation of the complement source with the test sera, is a measure of the amount of complement fixed or consumed by something in the test sera—presumably complexes composed of immunoglobulins that have the ability to fix complement (primarily IgG_1, IgG_3 and IgM). Sera from patients with JRA had a significantly (p less than .001) increased complement consumption when compared to hospitalized pediatric controls who had no evidence of rheumatoid disease.[32] In a subsequent study, values from children with JRA divided into defined subgroups, were correlated with the patients' clinical ratings made on the basis of clinical appearance alone (independent of *any* other laboratory data). It was found that all those with JRA had increased complement consumption above that of their age-matched normal outpatient controls (p less than .01). Furthermore, disease activity was correlated with complement consumption in those who had rheumatoid factor-negative polyarticular JRA (p less than .01) (Table I).[33] Sera of children with rheumatoid factor-positive disease had a complement consumption that fluctuated above normal but still correlated with variations in symptomatology.[33] In both rheumatoid factor-positive adults and children, the complement consumption observed was independent of the titer of rheumatoid factor.[31]

When longitudinal studies were performed in children with active polyarticular, rheumatoid factor-negative JRA over a four-year period, an increase in complement consumption appeared in most children prior to a relative fall in the total hemolytic complement and a rise in clinical activity. (L.M. Pachman, S. Baldwin, and M. Cobb, unpublished data.) The ability of the children's sera to activate the complement cascade was independent of the concentration of immunoglobulins at the time of testing.[32,33] Addition of exogenous IgG to either normal or JRA sera prior to heating at 56C for thirty minutes (to inactivate the endogenous complement) did not increase the amount of complement consumption, indicating that the assay detects *pre-formed* substance(s) present in the patients' sera rather than those that may have been induced during the heating step.[33] Inasmuch as a variety of substances such as C-reactive protein (CRP) activate the complement system by binding with C1q,[34] sera of patients with active JRA were

Table I
Complement Consumption by Sera of 89 Children With Rheumatoid Factor-Negative JRA

Group	N*	Mean Hemolysis Measured as O.D. − background	Standard Deviation	% C'C†	P values‡ vs Normal	vs Active
Normal	15	0.632	0.025	0	—	
Monoarticular JRA						
Active	8	0.544	0.065	15	less than 0.01	—
Borderline	5	0.479	0.038	18	less than 0.01	n.s.§
Inactive	6	0.492	0.078	19	less than 0.01	n.s.
Pauciarticular JRA						
Active	12	0.465	0.091	22	much less than 0.01	—
Borderline	10	0.507	0.072	14	much less than 0.01	n.s.
Inactive	10	0.491	0.063	20	much less than 0.01	n.s.
Polyarticular JRA						
Active	12	0.430	0.074	31	much less than 0.01	—
Borderline	12	0.522	0.061	15	much less than 0.01	<.01
Inactive	14	0.522	0.068	15	much less than 0.01	<.01

*One sample per patient

†Mean C'C = 100 − $\dfrac{\text{Hemolysis (O.D.)} - \text{background (O.D.)}}{\text{O.D. of maximum C'lysis}}$

‡Wilcoxon's test
§Not significant

tested for correlations with CRP, erythrocyte sedimentation rate (ESR), and complement consumption. The three functions varied independently: patients with elevated ESR and CRP had an elevated complement consumption as did most children with active disease and normal levels of CRP and ESR.

The nature of the presumed complexes in sera of patients with JRA remains to be proved and it is expected that there may be a heterogeneity in their composition as well.

Complement Fragments as Soluble Mediators of Inflammation

The third component of complement, C3, can be degraded into several fragments, the specific activity of each a subject of current investigation.[8] It is well recognized that in addition to being the most abundant component of complement in sera, C3 can be cleaved into its active fragments as a consequence of factors which activate either the direct or the alternate pathway. In addition, several noncomplement related proteolytic enzymes, some of which are cellular in origin, can directly cleave C3, the most ubiquitous of these being plasmin, thrombin, and trypsin.

Cleavage of C3 results in the formation of C3a, a very basic low molecular weight protein which is chemotactic for polymorphonuclear cells (PMNs) and monocytes. Depending on the condition of cleavage C3a retains its ability to contract smooth muscle (anaphylatoxinlike activity).[35]

The remainder of the digest C3b (which in itself is subsequently degraded into C3c and C3d) has a variety of effects. It can attach via a stable binding site to the membrane C3b receptor (immune adherence receptor), thus stimulating such cellular activity as monocyte phagocytosis and direct cytolysis. In addition, C3b is required for alternate pathway function. Other alternate pathway components can also affect a variety of cells: for example, factor B is secreted by macrophages and a cleavage product of factor B, Bb, can inhibit macrophage migration when added to C3b.[36] These cleavage products can also induce rapid macrophage membrane spreading.[37] Assays for C3d as a breakdown product of C3b have been widely used to provide evidence of complement activation, and it is known that cells have C3d receptors which can bind to C3b as well. Another fragment of C3, which is part of the C3c component has recently been isolated. This low molecular weight compound, C3e, can mobilize leukocytes from the bone marrow for a two-hour period and induces increased vascular permeability when injected intradermally.[38]

Other complement fragments can also attract inflammatory cells. C5a, a cleavage product of C5, is found in rheumatoid synovial fluid and is chemotactic for both polymorphonuclear cells and monocytes.[39] A chemotactic factor from normal human eosinophils, SECA, has been obtained from the sera of both rheumatoid factor-positive and -negative children with JRA and may be identical to C5a in structure.[40]

Recent assays of breakdown products of C3, C4 and properdin factor B have been applied to synovial fluid of patients with rheumatoid arthritis in order to determine evidence of complement activation. Increased levels of these breakdown products were found only in patients with rheumatoid arthritis whether rheumatoid factor-positive or -negative, but not in the synovial fluid obtained from patients with osteoarthritis.[41]

PHAGOCYTE FUNCTION IN JRA

Chemotaxis

Generation of neutrophil chemotactic factors may be accomplished by several pathways. It has been postulated by some that activation of Hageman factor by immune complexes results in the formation of chemotactic factors, kallikrein and plasminogen, both of which demonstrate chemotactic ability.[42,43] In addition, collagenase (a neutral protease produced by synovial cells and monocytes) as well as fibrin degradation products can act as chemotactic factors. As noted above, complement components, C3a[35] and C5a[39] as well as $C\overline{567}$[44] can be generated by appropriate stimulation of the complement cascade. IgE-dependent immune activation of mast cells and basophils can result in the release of eosinophil chemotactic factor of anaphylaxis (ECF-A).[45]

Each of the various chemotactic factors may have specific target cells. For example, C3a and C5a attract mononuclear leukocytes, eosinophils, and neutrophils with equivalent activity for each cell type.[46] Collagenase per se is strongly chemotactic for neutrophils but not for macrophages, while fibrin degradation products except fibrinogen, fibrin, and plasmin, attract neutrophils alone.[47] Finally, other cells may have products that are chemotactic for monocytes, such as the one derived from T lymphocytes.[48]

Very few studies have addressed the question of the ability of the phagocyte to respond to chemotactic factors in juvenile rheumatoid arthritis. In several studies chemotaxis of neutrophils from both adults with RA and children with seronegative JRA was significantly less than from normal controls.[49] There was no correlation between the chemotactic index and disease activity; salicylates did not alter chemotaxis. However, those patients with the lowest serum complement had the most impaired chemotaxis. Exposure of normal PMN's to isolated complexes also resulted in decreased PMN chemotaxis, implying that either the receptor for C3a was blocked or that the cells were unable to respond because of metabolic changes following phagocytosis.[49]

PMN chemotaxis can be mediated by rheumatoid factor via activation of the complement pathway.[50,51] Monocyte chemotaxis has been briefly reported to be abnormal in children with JRA who were treated with aspirin, but correlation with disease activity and therapy has not been demonstrated.[52]

The NBT test in JRA

Circulating soluble immune complexes may affect another test of phagocyte activation—the nitroblue tetrazolium test (NBT). Many observers have noted that the results of this test are elevated above normal in children with active JRA who are either rheumatoid factor-positive or -negative.[53] When the sera of children with active disease were incubated with normal polymorphonuclear cells, these normal leukocytes became NBT-positive suggesting stimulation of phagocytosis by some substance in the sera.[54,55] Addition of soluble artificial complexes could produce NBT-positive cells in vitro with maximum stimulation at the range of slight antigen excess (4 to 1).[54,56] In vivo studies in rabbits demonstrated that the NBT test became positive in the stage of early antibody formation and was maximal at equivalence but remained elevated.[54]

Phagocytosis and Rheumatoid Factor

Phagocytosis by synovial fluid leukocytes of IgG rheumatoid factor has been demonstrated with varying degrees of success using articular aspirates from rheumatoid factor-negative patients.[9-11] When synovial fluids from five patients with JRA were incubated with normal peripheral blood leukocytes, cytoplasmic inclusions of IgG were found in two using immunofluorescent techniques.[57] Recent experiments in which the leukocytes of patients with JRA were challenged with latex particles demonstrated less uptake than was found using cells and sera from normal controls; there was no correlation with the patients' levels of rheumatoid factor, suggesting that previous ingestion of IgG complexes may have rendered these cells refractory to further stimulation.[58]

Lysosomal enzyme release has been used as an indicator of phagocyte stimulation. The effect of the size of the aggregate on enzyme release has been extensively studied by Henson[59] who documented that soluble IgG complexes were less efficient than larger aggregates in causing lysosomal enzyme release from peripheral blood PMN's.[59] Cathepsins,[60] acid hydrolases,[61] and neutral proteases, have all been identified as a consequence of immune complex phagocyte interaction in rheumatoid arthritis, but very few studies have included material from patients with JRA.[60,61] Efforts to identify respiratory gas changes (pCO_2, pO_2, pH) in synovial fluid of patients with JRA (which might reflect the phagocyte metabolic activity of synovial fluid components) have not been found useful as indicators of disease activity.[62]

The composition as well as the solubility of the test complexes has a pronounced influence on the results obtained in a given assay. Using insoluble rheumatoid factor-IgG complexes, fresh serum was required to demonstrate activation of the human polymorphonuclear hexose monophosphate shunt and release of lysosomal β-glucuronidase.[63] Furthermore, previous exposure to large molecules of IgM-rheumatoid factor may impair complement mediated phagocytosis of a challenge particle by human PMN's.[64] Phagocytosis in vitro of soluble immune complexes may not be enhanced by serum and has been reported to be a function of cell concentration, the amount of immune complex present, the duration of incubation, and the amount of antigen in excess of equivalence.[65] Therefore the composition of the complex, its antigen antibody ratio, as well as its size, may play a role in stimulation of subsequent lysosomal enzyme release. In general it is thought that the sera of children with rheumatoid factor-negative JRA contain soluble immune complexes which are less efficient in complement fixation than insoluble ones.[66]

THE CLOTTING SYSTEM AND JRA

Hageman factor, the initial factor in the intrinsic pathway of coagulation, has been reported to be activated by immune complexes. The resulting components interact with prekallikrein, creating kallikrein which is chemotactic for neutrophils.[42] Kallikrein, in addition, cleaves bradykinin from kininigen. Bradykinin can elicit edema for a short period of time. The interrelationship between the clotting system and the complement system at various steps is intricate and has recently been reviewed.[67] For example, Hageman factor can activate C1q via plasmin which also splits C3a from C3. In addition plasmin can activate the C$\overline{567}$ complex. Some rheumatoid factor immunoglobulins when mixed with IgG release kinin but this step is thought to be dependent on the presence of Hageman factor.[68] Some controversy surrounds this issue in that Cochrane et al. were not able to reproduce these results.[69] There may be several other interactions between the clotting and the complement system. For example, it has been proposed recently that properdin factor D of the alternate pathway may be a fragment of thrombin.[70] In addition, soluble complexes are more effective than insoluble ones in stimulating human leukocytes to release procoagulant activity,[71] but evidence of this activity in JRA has yet to be presented.

The presence of detectable levels of kinins in the fluids of the inflamed joints during the course of rheumatoid arthritis suggests that they may play a role in the pathogenesis of the immune complex disease. It is possible, however, that immune complexes may activate kinin formation directly and may proceed by a pathway independent of Hageman factor. For example, RA has been documented in a person with Hageman trait, suggesting that a non-Hageman factor pathway must exist to enable this release of kinin.[72] However, further evidence is needed from synovial fluid of children with JRA. No increase in kininogen was found in the fluid of joints from rheumatoid factor-negative JRA.[20]

PROSTAGLANDINS

Synthesis of Prostaglandins

Within the past few years a new area of research, the structure and function of prostaglandins, has emerged. These substances can be classified among the soluble mediators of inflammation. Furthermore, their synthesis is blocked by drugs commonly used in rheumatology, of which salicylate, the drug of choice for most children with JRA, and indomethacin are the best known examples. A symposium compiling some of the voluminous work in this area has recently been published.[73]

The major evidence that prostaglandins function as a soluble mediator of inflammation has been reviewed by Vane.[74] The precise mechanism by which prostaglandin synthesis is initiated is not known, but a variety of stimuli such as bradykinin and thrombin can provoke cell lines to initiate prostaglandin synthesis upon exposure. The primary prostaglandins, PgE_2 and PgF_2 and PgD_2, are formed by a cyclooxygenase acting on arachidonic acid (Figure 1). The transient cyclic endoperoxide intermediates, 15-hydroperoxy PgE_2 and PgH_2, may then end in one of three pathways:

(1) 15-hydroperoxy PgE$_2$ and PgH$_2$ can be isomerized to PgE$_2$ and/or PgD$_2$, or reduced to PgF$_2\alpha$; (2) platelets can form thromboxane A$_2$ via thromboxane synthetase with subsequent reduction of thromboxane B$_2$; or (3) prostaglandin E$_2$ can be produced via prostacylcin synthetase located in arterial lining cells. It is believed that the release of arachidonic acid from membrane phosolipid is the rate-limiting step in prostaglandin synthesis.

Cells do not store prostaglandin. Therefore release is dependent upon active synthesis, although probably only messenger RNA is needed. Synthesis of prostaglandins is effected by enzymes associated with the microsomal fractions of the cell and they are released when the membranes are distorted. In general the prostaglandins exert a maximal effect at the site of synthesis, probably mediating their action by controlling intracellular cyclic nucleotide levels: exogenous prostaglandins either increase or decrease intracellular adenosine cyclic 3′,5′ monophosphate (AMP), depending on the specific tissue under study. Aspirinlike drugs inhibit the synthesis and release of prostaglandins but do not reduce the inflammatory effects of injected prostaglandins either for pain or for inflammation.

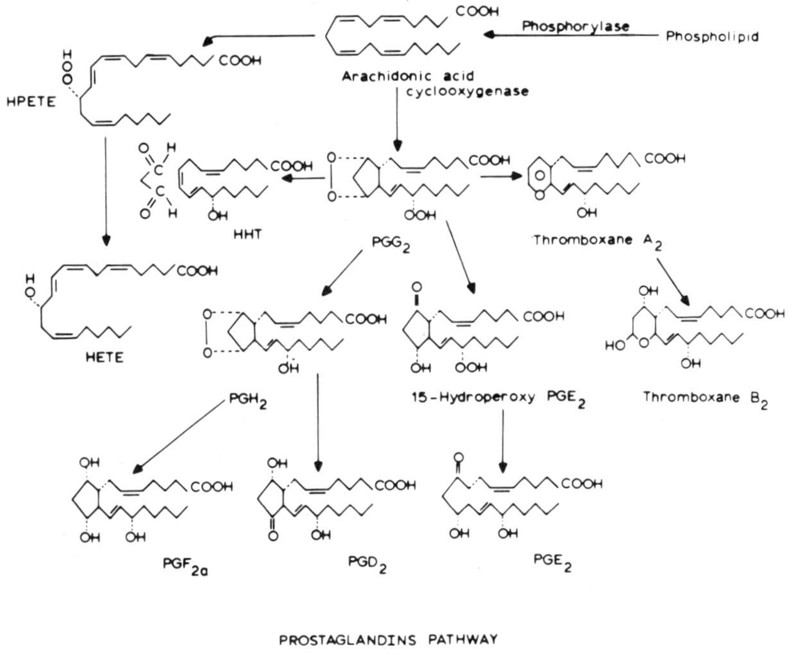

PROSTAGLANDINS PATHWAY

Figure 1. General outline of prostaglandins synthesis and structure. Synthesis of specific compounds is influenced by type of cell and microenvironmental conditions.

There are at least two components of discomfort of arthritis, the inflammatory process itself, and the perception of pain that is stimulated. The aspirinlike drugs are effective against local prostaglandin release rather than pain fiber stimulation, hence they act near or at the site of pain. Other soluble mediators of inflammation, i.e., bradykinin or rabbit aorta-contracting substance (thromboxane A_2) may act to stimulate prostaglandin release, and it is possible that increased local concentration of PgE_1 may sensitize the afferent nerve ending directly. The unstable intermediates, cyclic endoperoxides, may be even more potent than the end product in producing pain, but they too are reduced in the presence of aspirinlike drugs.[75]

Prostaglandins and Inflammation

Prostaglandins are released by many types of inflammatory stimuli such as histamine, bradykinin, and SRSA. In addition to pain, PgE_1 and PgE_2 can cause erythema and contribute to increased vascular permeability and edema as well as to hyperalgesia.[76] The most common prostaglandin found in inflammation is PgE_2 which is somewhat chemotactic for PMNs. However, during phagocytosis PMNs release PgE_1 which is both inflammatory and markedly chemotactic for yet other polymorphonuclear cells, thus perpetuating the cycle. In chronic inflammatory states, such as uveitis in a rabbit or rheumatoid arthritis in man, the major prostaglandin found at the inflammatory site is PgE_1 and it is associated with increased accummulation of polymorphonuclear cells.[77]

Human polymorphonuclear cells release other enzymes, for example, collagenase which is operative at both neutral and alkaline pH, as well as PgE_1 and PgE_2 as noted above.[78] Prostaglandins and agents which result in higher levels of intracellular cyclic AMP inhibit the release of lysosomal enzymes from human polymorphonuclear cells[79] and also inhibit chemotaxis.[80]

Prostaglandins and the Immune System

Analysis of synovial fluid obtained from patients with rheumatoid arthritis has demonstrated predominately PgE_1 and small amounts of $PgF_2\alpha$,[81] and their synthesis by synovial cells in vitro has been documented.[82] Cultures of rheumatoid synovia also produce collagenase, suggesting that these substances may play a central role in the pathogenesis of rheumatoid arthritis.[83] The adherent mononuclear cells release PgE_1 and this synthesis is inhibited by indomethacin while collagenase synthesis is unaffected. Furthermore, in vitro studies demonstrate that supernatant fluid from a phytohemagglutinin (PHA) stimulated nonadherent mononuclear cell culture activated adherent synovial cells to produce both collagenase and PgE_2, thus suggesting a regulatory role for lymphoid cells.[84] In other studies of synovial cultures, connective tissue-activating peptide (CTAP) stimulation was potentiated by prostaglandins, and hyaluronic acid synthesis was enhanced.[85]

The relationship of prostaglandins to the immune system has been the subject of investigation in several laboratories. Prostaglandins have been thought to inhibit both B-lymphocyte activity and T lymphocytes as a function of increased intracellular cyclic AMP,[86] but further studies may need to be performed using a more physiologic dosage range.[87] Prostaglandins diminish PHA reactivity (a T lymphocyte response) and appear to inhibit the production of lymphokines such as macrophage migration inhibition factor[88] as well as in vivo and in vitro autoimmunity.[89]

Therefore prostaglandins are not only produced by the cellular components of the immune system, but these cells themselves are susceptible to the action of prostaglandins, suggesting that prostaglandins may play a central role as regulators of the immune response.[90] One current theory of the pathogenesis of rheumatoid arthritis suggests that there may be a decreased susceptibility of lymphocytes from patients with this disease to control by local PgE_1, thus impairing a feedback limitation of the release of lymphokines which perpetuate the inflammatory response.[91] The most recent investigations concern the relationship of prostaglandin derivatives, endoperoxides and thromboxane, and the clotting mechanism.[92]

The relationship of the therapeutic agent to prostaglandin synthesis is of importance. The clinical effects of aspirinlike drugs appear to be direct correlates of their anticyclooxygenase activity. Noninflammatory agents such as morphine and antihistamines do not inhibit prostaglandin synthesis nor do steroidal antiinflammatory drugs, suggesting that these agents have different sites of action in ameliorating the inflammatory process. When aspirin is given in therapeutic doses, the free (nonprotein-bound) concentration is sufficient to inhibit prostaglandin biosynthesis efficiently.

The Effect of a Prostaglandin Inhibitor (Salicylate) in JRA

Specific investigation of prostaglandin synthesis and function has not been accomplished in the juvenile patient. Therefore the evidence of the mechanism of action of salicylate must be derived from observations in the clinical area, both in vivo and in vitro. One of the major immunoregulatory roles of salicylate has been postulated to be the suppressive action on T lymphocyte responses to mitogens and anti-gens.[93] This inhibitory effect is rapidly reversible in vitro, and is corre-lated with the dosage of salicylate present as well as with another selective effect of salicylate—uncoupling of oxidative phosphorylation. IgM synthesis by isolated spleen cells in vitro was markedly reduced by salicylate whereas IgG synthesis was found to be relatively unim-paired.[94] It was speculated that just as there is variability in the species and cell source of cyclooxygenase sensitivity to salicylate, so variation in cellular dependence on oxidative phosphorylation might be critical to other antiinflammatory actions of this drug.

A few in vitro studies of the effect of salicylate on phagocyte function have been performed. Salicylate added in appropriate concen-trations (20mg/dl) to assays of phagocytic function using opsonic anti-body and type 12, group A *beta*-hemolytic streptococci or to staph-ylococci did not impair uptake or killing by normal human PMNs, indicating that this critical function is probably intact in the treated patient.[95] Salicylate had no effect when particles were added to stimu-late NBT dye reduction by human leukocytes. The concentration of salicylate achieved in the sera in the usual course of therapy did not inhibit the complement consumption assay; a marked interference was seen at three times this concentration. The few in vivo investigations which have been performed raise some question concerning the precise role of salicylate in altering immune function in JRA.

Studies of children with JRA or rheumatic fever receiving therapeutic doses of salicylate (blood level greater than 20mg/dl) did not demonstrate impairment of the normal sequence of events in the inflammatory response using the Rebuck skin window technique.[95] When peripheral lymphocytes from five children with rheumatoid factor-negative polyarticular JRA were stimulated with increasing con-centrations of mitogens (PHA or Conconavalin A) before and after six weeks of salicylate therapy, no significant difference in cellular re-sponse was noted (L.M. Pachman, M.D. Mikus and M. Cobb, unpub-lished observations). Recent reports of skin testing in treated and untreated adult volunteers suggest that after five days of therapeutic doses of salicylate there was no alteration in skin test reactivity, lymphocyte proliferation, or T cell number.[96] Further information about the effects of salicylate on the immune response in JRA is needed before conclusions about its role in vivo can be formulated.

SUMMARY

Soluble mediators of inflammation include humoral factors and cellular products. Evidence from available studies utilizing data from patients with JRA indicates that the direct pathway of complement is activated intraarticularly and that substances, presumed to be complexes, are present in JRA sera which also activate complement. The presence of kinins in the synovial fluid suggests participation in the clotting system but further evaluation is needed. Immune complexes affect phagocyte function and there is some evidence that phagocyte function has in fact been altered in JRA. It is not known if the response of cells to, or their production of, prostaglandins, is age-related. The precise role of salicylate, a prostaglandin inhibitor, in altering the immune response in JRA remains to be documented. It is expected that further definition of the heterogenous group of patients with juvenile rheumatoid arthritis, as well as increased data concerning the pharmacological effects of various drugs effective in therapy, will give insight into the pathophysiology of JRA.

Editor's note: Dr. Pachman is apparently more convinced than I of the ubiquity of antigen-antibody complexes in JRA (see Chapter 4). This is a point of healthy controversy, since this is the most important current question regarding pathogenesis and classification of JRA.

REFERENCES

1. Wright, V. The syndrome of seronegative spondarthritis. Edited by D.C. Dumonde. In *Infection and Immunity in the Rheumatic Diseases*. Oxford and Edinburgh: Blackwell Scientific, 1974, pp. 319–25.

2. Gabay, R., Zubler, R.H., Nydegger, U.E., and Lambert, P.H. Immune complexes and complement catabolism in ankylosing spondylitis. *Arthritis Rheum*. 20:913–16, 1977.

3. Hedberg, H. The depressed synovial complement in adult and juvenile rheumatoid arthritis. *Acta Rheum Scand*. 10:109–27, 1964.

4. Hedberg, H. The total complement activity of synovial fluid in juvenile forms of arthritis. *Acta Rheum Scand*. 17:279–85, 1971.

5. Bianco, N.E., Panush, R.S., Stillman, J.S., and Schur, P.H. Immunologic studies of juvenile rheumatoid arthritis. *Arthritis Rheum*. 14:685–96, 1971.

6. Ruddy, S., Matsuura, M., Stillman, J.S., and Austen, K.F. Complement component activities in serum and synovial fluid from patients with juvenile rheumatoid arthritis. Edited by W. Muller, H.G. Harwerth, and K. Fehr. In *Rheumatoid Arthritis*. London and New York: Academic Press, 1971, pp. 397–409.

7. Schur, P.H., Britton, M.C., Franco, A.E. et al. Rheumatoid synovitis: complement and immune complexes. *Rheumatology*. 6:34–42, 1975.

8. Muller-Eberhard, H.J. The serum complement system. Edited by P.A. Miescher, and H.J. Muller-Eberhard. In *Textbook of Immunopathology*. New York: Grune and Stratton, 1976, pp. 45–73.

9. Fish, A.J., Michael, A.F., Gewurz, H., and Good, R.A. Immunopathologic changes in rheumatoid arthritis synovium. *Arthritis Rheum*. 9:267–80, 1966.

78

10. Cats, A., Lafeber, G.J.M., and Klein, F. Immunoglobulin phagocytosis by granulocytes from sera and synovial fluids in various rheumatoid and nonrheumatoid diseases. *Ann Rheum Dis*. 34:146–55, 1975.

11. Britton, M.C., and Schur, P.H. The complement system in rheumatoid synovitis. II. Intracytoplasmic inclusions of immunoglobulins and complement. *Arthritis Rheum*. 14:87–95, 1971.

12. Hollander, J.L., McCarty, D.J., Astorga, G., and Castro-Murillo, E. Studies on the pathogenesis of rheumatoid joint inflammation. I. The "R.A. cell" and a working hypothesis. *Ann Int Med*. 62:271–80, 1965.

13. Pekin, T.J., and Zvaifler, N.J. Hemolytic complement in synovial fluid. *J Clin Invest*. 43:1372–82, 1964.

14. Hannestad, K. Presence of aggregated γG-globulin in certain rheumatoid synovial effusions. *Clin Exp Immunol*. 2:511–29, 1967.

15. Pope, R.M., Teller, D.C., and Mannik, M. The molecular basis of self-association of IgG rheumatoid factors. *J Immunol*. 115:365–73, 1975.

16. Natvig, J.B., Munthe, E., and Pahle, J. Evidence for intracellular complement-fixing complexes of IgG rheumatoid factor in rheumatoid plasma cells. *Rheumatology*. 6:167–76, 1975.

17. Winchester, R.J., Agnello, V., and Kunkel, H.G. The joint-fluid γG-globulin complexes and their relationship to intraarticular complement diminution. *Ann NY Acad Sci*. 168:195–203, 1969.

18. Lambert, P.H., Nydegger, U.E., Perrin, L.H. et al. Complement activation in seropositive and seronegative rheumatoid arthritis. *Rheumatology*. 6:52–9, 1975.

19. Zvaifler, N.J. Breakdown products of C'3 in human synovial fluids. *J Clin Invest*. 48:1532–42, 1969.

20. Rynes, R.I., Ruddy, S., Spragg, J. et al. Intraarticular activation of the complement system in patients with juvenile rheumatoid arthritis. *Arthritis Rheum*. 19:161–8, 1976.

21. Donde, R., Permin, H., Juhl, F. et al. Immune deposits in the dermoepidermal junction in rheumatoid arthritis. *Scand J Rheumatol*. 6:57–61, 1977.

22. Vaughan, J.H., Bayles, T.B., and Favour, C.B. Serum complement in rheumatoid arthritis. *Am J Med Sci*. 222:186–192, 1951.

23. Wedgwood, R.J.P., and Janeway, C.A. Serum complement in children with "collagen diseases." *Pediatrics*. 11:569–80, 1953.

24. Høyeraal, H.M., and Mellbye, O.J. High levels of serum complement factors in juvenile rheumatoid arthritis. *Ann Rheum Dis*. 33:243–7, 1974.

25. Norman, M.E., Gall, E.P., Taylor, A. et al. Serum complement profiles in infants and children. *J Pediatr*. 87:912–16, 1975.

26. Masi, M., and Vivarelli, F. I livelli sierici di C'3 (β-1C/β–1-A globulina) in soggetti normali nelle varie eta' pediatriche. *Clin Pediatr*. (Bologna) 53:167–74, 1971.

27. Norman, M.E., Taylor, A., Green, P. et al. Studies of the alternative complement pathway (AP) in normal children. *J Immunol*. 1978. (In press)

28. Gutowska-Grzegorczyk, G., and Baum, J. Serum immunoglobulin and complement interrelationships in juvenile rheumatoid arthritis. *J Rheumatol*. 4:179–85, 1977.

29. Rudnicki, R.D., Ruderman, M., Scull, E. et al. Clinical features and serologic abnormalities in juvenile rheumatoid arthritis. *Arthritis Rheum*. 17:1007–15, 1974.

30. Goel, K.M., Logan, R.W., Barnard, W.P., and Shanks, R.A. Serum immunoglobulin and $\beta 1c/\beta 1A$ globulin concentrations in juvenile rheumatoid arthritis. *Ann Rheum Dis.* 33:35–8, 1974.

31. Pachman, L.M., Baldwin, S.M., and Gaekwar, S.M. Anticomplementary activity of sera from patients with juvenile rheumatoid arthritis (JRA), rheumatoid arthritis (RA), systemic lupus erythematosus (SLE) and normal controls, abstracted. *Pediatr Res.* 9:333, 1975.

32. Pachman, L.M., and Baldwin, S.M. Assays of complement in polyarticular juvenile rheumatoid arthritis. *Arthritis Rheum.* 20 (suppl):467–70, 1977.

33. Pachman, L.M., Mikus, M.D., and Baldwin, S.M. The effect of normal human sera (NHS) on complement consumption (CC) by immune serum globulin (ISG) or isolated human IgG (IgG), abstracted. *Pediatr Res.* 11:491, 1977.

34. Kaplan, M.H., and Volanakis, J.E. Interaction of C-reactive protein complexes with the complement system. *J Immunol.* 112:2135–47, 1974.

35. Bokisch, V.A., Muller-Eberhard, H.J., and Cochrane, C.G. Isolation of a fragment (C_3a) of the third component of human complement containing anaphylatoxin and chemotactic activity and description of an anaphylatoxin inactivator of human serum. *J Exp Med.* 129:1109–29, 1969.

36. Bianco, C., Goetz, O., and Cohn, Z.A. Regulation of macrophage motility by components of the complement system. *J Immunol.* 1978. (In press)

37. Goetz, O., Bianco, C., and Cohn, Z.A. The induction of macrophage spreading by Factor B of the properdin system. *J Immunol.* 1978. (In press)

38. Ghebrehiwet, B., and Muller-Eberhard, H.J. Description of an acidic fragment (C_3e) of human C_3 having leukocytosis-producing activity. *J Immunol.* 1978. (In press)

39. Ward, P.A. Complement-dependent phlogistic factors in rheumatoid synovial fluids. *Ann NY Acad Sci.* 256:169–76, 1975.

40. Robinson, L.D., and Miller, M.E. SECA, a new mediator of the human eosinophil response. *J Allergy Clin Immunol.* 56:317–22, 1975.

41. Perrin, L.H., Nydegger, U.E., Zubler, R.H. et al. Correlation between levels of breakdown products of C_3, C_4 and properdin factor B in synovial fluids from patients with rheumatoid arthritis. *Arthritis Rheum.* 20:647–52, 1977.

42. Kaplan, A.P., Kay, A.B., and Austen, K.F. A prealbumin activator of prekallikrein. III. Appearance of chemotactic activity for human neutrophils by the conversion of human prekallikrein to kallikrein. *J Exp Med.* 135:81–97, 1972.

43. Kaplan, A.P., Goetzl, E.J., and Austen, K.F. The fibrinolytic pathway of human plasma. II. The generation of chemotactic activity by activation of plasminogen proactivator. *J Clin Invest.* 52:2591–5, 1973.

44. Lachman, P.J., Kay, A.B., and Thompson, R.A. The chemotactic activity for neutrophil and eosinophil leukocytes of the trimolecular complex of the fifth, sixth, and seventh components of human complement (C567) prepared in free solution by the "reactive lysis" procedure. *Immunology.* 19:895–9, 1970.

45. Kay, A.B., Stechschulte, D.J., and Austen, K.F. An eosinophil leukocyte chemotactic factor of anaphylaxis. *J Exp Med.* 133:602–19, 1971.

46. Goetzl, E.J. Plasma and cell-derived inhibitors of human neutrophil chemotaxis. *Ann NY Acad Sci.* 256:210–21, 1975.

47. Stecer, V.J. The chemotaxis of selected cell types to connective tissue degradation products. *Ann NY Acad Sci.* 256:177–89, 1975.

48. Altman, L.C., Wahl, S.M., Kirchner, H. et al. Comparative studies of a lymphokine chemotactic for mononuclear leukocytes in humans, guinea pigs and chickens. *Proceedings of the Eighth Leucocyte Culture Conference.* London and New York: Academic Press, 1974, pp. 395–400.

49. Mowat, A.G., and Baum, J. Chemotaxis of polymorphonuclear leukocytes from patients with rheumatoid arthritis. *J Clin Invest.* 50:2541–9, 1971.

50. Stojan, B., Borel, J.F., and Loewi, G. Chemotactic effect of joint effusions. *Ann Rheum Dis.* 33:425–7, 1974.

51. Borel, J.F., Sorkin, E., and Loewi, G. Neutrophil chemotaxis mediated by rheumatoid factor. *Immunology.* 21:165–7, 1971.

52. Fischer, T.J., Klein, R.B., Borut, T.C. et al. Monocyte chemotaxis in health and disease, abstracted. *Pediatr Res.* 11:486, 1977.

53. Feigin, R.D., Shackleford, P.D., Choi, S.C. et al. Nitroblue tetrazolium dye test as an aid in the differential diagnosis of febrile disorders. *J Pediatr.* 78:230–7, 1971.

54. Pachman, L.M., Jayanetra, P., and Rothberg, R.M. Rheumatoid sera and soluble complexes: nitroblue tetrazolium dye test and hexose monophosphate shunt activation. *Pediatrics.* 52:823–30, 1973.

55. John, M., and Oppermann, J. The nitroblue tetrazolium test in juvenile rheumatoid arthritis and the stimulation of granulocytes by patients' sera. *Scand J Rheumatol.* 6:81–6, 1977.

56. Hawkins, D., and Peeters, S. The response of polymorphonuclear leukocytes to immune complexes in vitro. *Lab Invest.* 24:483–91, 1971.

57. Hurd, E.R., LoSpalluto, J., and Ziff, M. Formation of leukocyte inclusions in normal polymorphonuclear cells incubated with synovial fluid. *Arthritis Rheum.* 13:724–33, 1970.

58. Coberand, J., Amigues, H., de Larrard, B., and Pradere, J. Neutrophil function in rheumatoid arthritis. *Scand J Rheumatol.* 6:49–52, 1977.

59. Henson, P.M. Mechanisms of release of granule enzymes from human neutrophils phagocytosing aggregated immunoglobulin. An electron microscopic study. *Arthritis Rheum.* 16:208–16, 1973.

60. Oronsky, A.R., and Perper, R.J. Connective tissue degrading enzymes of human leukocytes. *Ann NY Acad Sci.* 256:233–53, 1975.

61. Weissman, G., Zurier, R.B., Spieler, P.J., and Goldstein, I.M. Mechanisms of lysosomal enzyme release from leukocytes exposed to immune complexes and other particles. *J Exp Med.* 134:149s–65s, 1971.

62. Goetzl, E.J., Rynes, R.I., and Stillman, J.S. Abnormalities of respiratory gases in synovial fluid of patients with juvenile rheumatoid arthritis. *Arthritis Rheum.* 17:450–4, 1974.

63. Turner, R., Collins, R., Stott, K. et al. Immunoglobulin G complex interactions with rheumatoid factor and neutrophils $^{51}CrCl_3$ labeling and $^{14}CO_2$ hexose monophosphate shunt studies. *J Rheumatol.* 3:329–36, 1976.

64. McDuffie, F.C., and Brumfield, H.W. Effect of rheumatoid factor on complement-mediated phagocytosis. *J Clin Invest.* 51:3007–13, 1972.

65. Ward, P.A., and Zvaifler, N.J. Quantitative phagocytosis by neutrophils. I. A new method with immune complexes. *J Immunol.* 111:1771–6, 1973.

66. Lightfoot, R.W., Drusin, R.E., and Christian, C.L. Properties of soluble immune complexes. *J Immunol.* 105:1493–1500, 1970.

67. Zimmerman, T.S., Fierer, J., and Rothbergerer, H. Blood coagulation and the inflammatory response. *Sem Hematol.* 14:391–408, 1977.

68. Eisen, V., and Smith, H.G. Plasma kinin formation by complexes of aggregated γ-globulin and serum proteins. *Br J Exp Path.* 51:328–31, 1970.

69. Cochrane, C.G., Wuepper, K.D., Aiken, B.S. et al. The interaction of Hageman factor and immune complexes. *J Clin Invest.* 51:2736–45, 1972.

70. Davis, A.E., Rosenberg, R.D., Fenton, J.W. et al. Is factor D of the alternate pathway a fragment of thrombin? *J Immunol.* 1978. (In press)

71. Rothbergerer, H., Zimmerman, T.S., Spiegelberg, H.L., and Vaughan, J.H. Leukocyte procoagulant activity. *J Clin Invest.* 59:549–57, 1977.

72. Donaldson, V.H., Glueck, H.I., and Fleming, T. Rheumatoid arthritis in a patient with Hageman trait. *N Engl J Med.* 286:528–30, 1972.

73. Robinson, H.J., and Vane, J.R., eds. *Prostaglandin Synthetase Inhibitors.* New York: Raven Press, 1974.

74. Vane, J.R. Mode of action of aspirin and similar compounds. Edited by H.J. Robinson and J.R. Vane. In *Prostaglandin Synthetase Inhibitors.* New York: Raven Press, 1974, pp. 155–63.

75. Ferreira, S.H., Moncada, S., and Vane, J.R. Prostaglandins and signs and symptoms of inflammation. Edited by H.J. Robinson and J.R. Vane. In *Prostaglandin Synthetase Inhibitors.* New York: Raven Press, 1974, pp. 175–87.

76. Flower, R.J. The role of prostaglandins in inflammatory reactions. *Arch Pharmacol.* 297:s77–s79, 1977.

77. Zurier, R.B., and Sayadoff, D.M. Release of prostaglandins from human polymorphonuclear leukocytes. *Inflammation.* 1:93–101, 1975.

78. Lazarus, G.S., Brown, R.S., Daniel, J.R., and Fullmer, H.M. Human granulocyte collagenase. *Science.* 159:1483–5, 1968.

79. Zurier, R.B., Hoffstein, A., and Weissmann, G. Mechanisms of lysosomal enzyme release from human leukocytes. *J Cell Biol.* 58:27–41, 1973.

80. Hill, H.R., Estenson, R.D., Quie, P.G. et al. Modulation of human neutrophilic chemotactic response by cyclic 3'5' guanosine monophosphate and cyclic 3'5' adenosine monophosphate. *Metabolism.* 24:447–50, 1975.

81. Higgs, G.A., Vane, J.R., Hart, F.D., and Wojtulewski, J.A. Effects of antiinflammatory drugs on prostaglandins in rheumatoid arthritis. Edited by H.J. Robinson, and J.R. Vane. in *Prostaglandin Synthetase Inhibitors.* New York: Raven Press, 1974, pp. 165–73.

82. Crook, D., and Collins, A.J. Prostaglandin synthetase activity from human rheumatoid synovial tissue and its inhibition by nonsteroidal anti-inflammatory drugs. *Prostaglandins.* 9:857–65, 1975.

83. Krane, S.M. Collagenase production by human synovial tissues. *Ann NY Acad Sci.* 256:289–303, 1975.

84. Dayer, J.M., Robinson, D.R., and Krane, S.M. Prostaglandin production by rheumatoid synovial cells. Stimulation by a factor from human mononuclear cells. *J Exp Med.* 145:1399–1404, 1977.

85. Castor, C.W. Connective tissue activation. VII. Evidence supporting a role for prostaglandins and cyclic nucleotides. *J Lab Clin Med.* 85:392–404, 1975.

86. Bourne, H.R., Lichtenstein, L.M., Melmon, K.L. et al. Modulation of inflammation and immunity by cyclic AMP. *Science.* 184:19–28, 1974.

87. Berenbaum, M.C., Purves, E.C., and Addison, I.E. Intercellular immunological controls and modulation of cyclic AMP levels. Some doubts. *Immunology*. 30:815–23, 1976.

88. Gordon, D., Bray, M.A., and Morley, J. Control of lymphokine secretion by prostaglandins. *Nature*. 262:815–23, 1976.

89. Strom, T.B., Carpenter, C.B., Cragoe, E.J. et al. Suppression of in vivo and in vitro alloimmunity by prostaglandins. *Transplant Proc*. 9:1075–9, 1977.

90. Pelus, L.M., and Strausser, H.R. Prostaglandins and the immune response. *Life Sci*. 20:903–14, 1977.

91. Morley, J. Prostaglandins and lymphokines in arthritis. *Prostaglandins*. 8:315–26, 1974.

92. Marx, J.L. Blood clotting: the role of the prostaglandins. *Science*. 196:1072–5, 1977.

93. Pachman, L.M., Esterly, N.B., and Peterson, R.D.A. The effect of salicylate in the metabolism of normal and stimulated human lymphocytes in vitro. *J Clin Invest*. 50:226–30, 1971.

94. Alm, C.V., and Pachman, L.M. The effects of sodium salicylate on the anamnestic immune response in vitro. *Experientia*. 27:924–5, 1971.

95. Pachman, L.M. The effect of salicylate on the function and metabolism of peripheral blood leukocytes, abstracted. *Fed Proc*. 29:492, 1970.

96. Duncan, M.W., Person, D.A., Rich, R.R., and Sharp, J.T. Aspirin and delayed type hypersensitivity. *Arthritis Rheum*. 20:1174–8, 1977.

7 The Pathology of Cartilage in Juvenile Rheumatoid Arthritis

J. Roger Hollister

Although the majority of descriptions of pathology of juvenile rheumatoid arthritis have focused on the synovial fluid and the synovium within joints, the changes of cartilage warrant analysis and understanding since they are often irreversible and productive of much of the morbidity in this disease. The chronic inflammatory lesions in the soft tissues of the joint are proliferative in nature and responsible for the acute symptomatology of pain and swelling of affected joints. From experimental studies and observations of patients with remitting rheumatoid arthritis, it is clear that these proliferative inflammatory changes are reversible and not responsible for ongoing symptoms if the inflammation abates. Unless there is damage to the hard tissues comprising articular cartilage, menisci, and ligaments, joint function can be restored if the inflammation subsides. On the other hand, if prolonged stretching of ligaments, degeneration of menisci, or erosion of articular cartilage and underlying bone has resulted from the longstanding inflammation, the patient may continue to experience pain and loss of function even after the acute phase of rheumatoid arthritis has subsided. It is not uncommon for patients with JRA to reach young

83

adulthood with very little continuing inflammation or proliferation of synovial tissue, but they continue to experience significant symptoms related to the irreversible changes in cartilaginous tissue. The most debilitating of these late symptoms appear to be due to destructive changes in articular cartilage which are similar to osteoarthritic symptoms in older persons. Changes in synovium and synovial fluid responsible for the damage to cartilaginous tissue will be described in this chapter.

PATHOLOGY OF SYNOVIUM

The pathologic changes in the soft tissue and fluid of rheumatoid joints begin as inflammation and progress to proliferation. Two studies of synovia from patients in the first few weeks to months of rheumatoid arthritis have indicated that inflammation begins around capillaries and venules in the subsynovium coincident with synovial effusion and joint swelling.[1,2] The initial perivascular infiltrate consists of polymorphonuclear leukocytes (PMNs) and lymphocytes. Thereafter the cellular infiltrate spreads throughout the synovium and subsynovium and changes to a more chronic cellular picture of plasma cells and macrophages. A proliferation of the synovial lining is coincident with inflammatory changes. Normal synovial lining is a thin membranous structure of one or two cells of thickness. In the presence of chronic inflammation the synovial lining cells proliferate manyfold and increase the lining thickness. Villi grow into the synovial space. The mechanism of this proliferation remains obscure, and only the temporal sequence in association with chronicity of inflammation in rheumatoid arthritis gives a clue as to its nature.[3]

The normal function of the synovial membrane appears to be disrupted in this proliferative process.[4] Besides the phagocytic ability of some of the cells, other cells in the normal membrane secrete hyaluronic acid which gives synovial fluid its unique characteristics of viscosity and lubrication. Synovial fluid is a transudate of serum with the exception of hyaluronic acid added by the synovial lining. In the course of JRA it changes to a thin nonviscid fluid with diminished content of hyaluronic acid, presumably because of altered function of the proliferative synovium. In addition synovial fluid becomes an exudate. Although the cellular infiltrate in the synovium becomes chronic in nature, synovial fluid maintains acute characteristics. PMNs comprise the majority of cells in the exudate which may contain 30,000 to 40,000 cells per cubic millimeter, approaching concentrations seen in bacterial sepsis. The remainder of cells are usually lymphocytes. Protein content of the exudative synovial fluid approaches that of serum. Proteins such as fibrin which are not found in normal fluid enter as a result of increased capillary permeability. There is an unusual lowering of synovial fluid glucose in JRA, apparently due to impaired transport from serum and not as previously thought, to consumption by metabolically active inflammatory cells. However, these alterations in synovium and synovial fluid which produce swelling, pain, and loss of function would not be expected to cause deformity or permanent disability unless the cartilaginous structures of the joint(s) are damaged in an irreparable manner.

PATHOLOGY OF CARTILAGE

In describing the pathology of cartilage we will be primarily concerned with articular cartilage since it has been the best studied of the intraarticular collagenous tissues and it is probable that the same sequence of events occurs in the ligaments and menisci of joints. Normal articular hyaline cartilage is composed of two different subunits. First, collagen fibrils are enmeshed in a matrix of unusual glycosaminoglycans containing keratin sulfate, chondroitin sulfate, and hyaluronic acid. Second, ground substance together with collagen gives articular cartilage its unique characteristics of resiliency, low friction, and the "shock absorber" function important in weight-bearing. Each of these two subunits has independent contributions to the overall function of the joint.[5]

The end stage of chronic inflammation is disintegration of the articular cartilage with exposure of underlying bone which may articulate with opposing bone. Increasing pain and limitation of function are produced by this extreme loss of joint integrity. Subluxing deformities in JRA joints are probably due to similar deterioration in the capsule and ligaments in and about joints, plus the resultant unopposed mechanical forces by the muscle operating them. Ulnar deviation of the metacarpalphalangeal joints of the hand is due to displacement of bones which are restrained by incompetent ligaments, with poorly articulating surfaces due to cartilage and bone erosion and muscular vectors in an ulnar direction. In retracing the events leading to this end point, one can gain insight into the mechanisms of joint damage and discern possibly reversible events which could lead to new types of therapy.

The earliest changes in articular cartilage appear to occur in the proteoglycans on the free surface.[6] These areas fail to stain with toluidine blue by light microscopy which is a characteristic of the highly negatively charged ground substance of normal cartilage. Electron microscopy reveals that there is fibrin adherent to the free surface, and the superficial layers now contain an abundance of amorphous material which is believed to be the degradation products of proteoglycans and cell organelles from either invading PMNs or dying chondrocytes.[7] These changes in articular cartilage are seen throughout the surface and are not restricted to the area covered by pannus. In vitro experimental studies have also shown similar changes in articular cartilage not in intimate contact with inflammatory cells, pannus, or bone marrow.[8]

The final common pathway of cartilage destruction appears to involve several enzymes originating from cells within joint tissue and fluid. These enzymes are best described by their separate substrates in articular cartilage. The ground substance or matrix which appears to be degraded earliest in the course of rheumatoid arthritis is digested by a variety of proteolytic enzymes present in synovial fluid, synovial tissue, invading polymorphonuclear leukocytes, and the chondrocytes of the articular cartilage itself.[9-11] The best purified and described enzymes are the cathepsin series which are acid proteolytic enzymes.[12-15] Cathepsin enzymes are capable of degrading protein backbone to which sulfated sugars are attached in the proteoglycans. However, there has been a major practical objection to a primary role for this enzyme as it is most active at pH5 and shows a 5- to 10-fold decrease in proteolytic activity as the pH of the reaction mixture approaches neutrality.[15] What investigations have been performed on the pH of synovial fluid, articular cartilage, and other points within the joint have indicated a range of 6.6 to 7.2.[13] It remains possible that intracellular lysosomal environment of phagocytic cells may have a pH in the acid range; then the cathepsin series would resume increased significance.

Less purified proteolytic enzymes for the proteoglycan substrate which are active at neutral pH have been extracted from synovium and inflammatory cells.[16-18] Beginning with the work of Ziff[19] and Weissman[20] considerable evidence demonstrates that these extracted enzymes are capable of digesting proteoglycans in solution or in native cartilage. As none of them has been purified to homogeneity, they remain a diverse group known as neutral proteases. A variety of other mechanisms for proteoglycan digestion have been described from such diverse sources as mitogen-stimulated lymphocytes, superoxide radicals in polymorphonuclear leukocytes, and the plasmin enzyme present in serum or synovial fluid.[21-23] It is impossible at this time to evaluate which enzyme series produces the major damage to articular cartilage ground substance.

The remarkable effectiveness of proteases was first demonstrated by Thomas who produced a complete collapse of ear cartilage in rabbit ears in vivo leading to a floppy-eared appearance.[24] This collapse was due to loss of proteoglycans but not collagen, demonstrated histochemically, and was fully reversible within four days after an intravenous injection of papain. With the restoration of matrix, the ear resumed its normal upright position. Therefore, not only are proteases most likely the initial enzyme system responsible for cartilage deterioration, but damage caused to proteoglycan ground substance may in fact be reversible at an early stage. The proteoglycan matrix is in fact quite active metabolically in contrast to the original evidence that it is an inert tissue. The half-life of turnover of proteoglycans has been estimated to be eight to 10 days.[25,26] In contrast, collagen fibers, the other subunit of articular cartilage have a very slow turnover rate. In both degenerative arthritis and rheumatoid arthritis it has been demonstrated that chondrocytes are metabolically more active and produce increased amounts of glycosaminoglycans; yet the degradation must be even more rapid as the net content of these substances is reduced in both conditions.[27] If enzymatic catabolism of proteoglycans can be interrupted, synthetic ability of chondrocytes might restore the integrity of cartilage.[24,28]

Collagen is also broken down by specific enzymes from several sources within the joints. Highly purified collagenase which splits the collagen molecule into smaller fragments has been isolated from inflammatory cells, synovium, synovial fluid, and articular cartilage itself.[29-31] Smaller digested collagen fragments appear to be substrates for other enzymes leading to total denaturation and solubilization of collagen. It is an attractive hypothesis that the early change in proteoglycan content of ground substance increases permeability of articular cartilage to collagenase enzymes which in turn cause further damage. The major theoretical problem with the collagenase system is existence of a number of potent inhibitors in vivo in alpha$_1$ and alpha$_2$ macroglobulins in serum and synovial fluid.[32] It is presently difficult to conceive of a dissociation of inhibitors from enzyme on the joint surface, except in the limited environment where pannus and articular cartilage are in such close proximity that inhibitors might be excluded.

The remarkable proliferative and destructive character of synovial pannus in rheumatoid arthritis is intimately linked to cartilage destruction. Pannus is a complex tissue having proliferative and hypertrophied synovial lining cells, an increase in tissue vascularity, and a variety of inflammatory cells including both neutrophils and mononuclear cells, in the subsynovium. Pannus originates from the synovial reflection over cartilage and begins a circumferential invasion of articular tissue and surrounding capsules and ligaments. Elegant electron microscopy of cartilage-pannus junction by Kobayashi and Ziff has demonstrated the invasive potential of pannus into cartilage with resulting dissolution of ground substance, collagen fibrils, and chondrocytes.[33] The intimate relationship between pannus and the underlying degenerating cartilage may provide an optimal environment for proteases and collagenases believed to be responsible for the final common pathway of cartilage destruction. In fact, collagenase has been localized to this junction with immunofluorescent techniques.[34] In vitro models have also demonstrated that the destruction of cartilage is markedly enhanced in cultures containing synovial cells or pannus.[35] The final proof that irreversible changes in cartilage are due to pannus comes from the original morphology of rheumatoid arthritis in that erosions in cartilage and bone actually begin at the circumference of the joint underlying invasive pannus. The stimulus for this invasive, inflammatory, destructive tissue in rheumatoid arthritis remains unknown.

ANTIGENS IN CARTILAGE

Whether cartilage is the passive target of destructive influences of rheumatoid arthritis or an active stimulant for prolonged inflammation poses an intriguing question. Considerable evidence has accrued that there are immune complexes in synovial fluid which are capable of activating complement and the subsequent inflammatory sequence. The antigenic component of these immune complexes remains elusive, and it remains possible that other structures within the joint may also be involved in initiation and prolongation of disease. Autoimmunity to cartilage has been proposed as one possible mechanism, but experimental support for this hypothesis has not been forthcoming.[36] In fact, antibodies to collagen appear to be ubiquitous in synovial fluid in a variety of inflammatory and noninflammatory lesions.[37] Other workers have attempted to define a putative antigen within the proteoglycan matrix,[38] but antibodies to these determinants have not been proven.

There is evidence in animal models of rheumatoid arthritis and correlative studies in the human disease suggesting that material which is not of cartilage origin may become trapped for long periods of time on the surface of cartilage. This phlogistic material may provide continued inflammatory stimulus for rheumatoid arthritis. In various experimental animals it is possible to produce an arthritis which is morphologically similar to rheumatoid arthritis.[39] Following systemic immunization of the animal injection of antigen into the joints will cause a synovitis which lasts many months and eventually develops into lymphoid nodules, pannus formation, and erosions very similar to those in rheumatoid arthritis. The incitement for this prolonged inflammation is formation of immune complexes between antigen and specific antibody in cartilaginous tissue within the joint. Shortly after injection antigen is cleared from the synovial fluid and tissue, and does not exist in these areas to promote long-term inflammation. On the other hand, binding of immune complexes in the outer five microns of cartilaginous tissue appears to sequester them away from normal host defenses.[40] The half-life of these bound immune complexes appears to parallel duration of the synovitis. Further support for this theory of pathogenesis has been gained from studies which indicate that these tissue-bound immune complexes are capable of generating chemotactic factors and fixing complement.[41] Chemotactic tissue-bound complexes offer an attractive explanation for production of an invasive pannus over the surface of articular cartilage. Correlative human studies have indicated that patients with rheumatoid arthritis have immunoglobulin and complement bound in the same areas of collagenous tissue.[42,43] Further studies are necessary in the human disease to recover immune complexes from cartilaginous tissue and to identify the responsible antigen.

CONCLUSIONS

In this chapter the mechanisms of cartilage destruction in rheumatoid arthritis have been reviewed. Given the fact that collagen has a low rate of turnover in articular cartilage and experimental evidence that newly synthesized collagen by chondrocytes in an inflammatory state is different from native articular cartilage collagen, it appears likely that damage produced by collagenolysis has reached a point of irreversibility in rheumatoid arthritis, yet loss of proteoglycan may be a reversible stage in the disease.[44] Data on JRA are very limited but suggest that growing cartilage of children over the femoral head is capable of regeneration.[45] Although the same degradative enzymatic processes may be responsible in JRA for destruction of joint articular cartilage, there may be an increased restorative capacity which should be taken advantage of in the future.

REFERENCES

1. Kulka, J.P., Bocking, D., Ropes, M.W., and Bauer, W. Early joint lesions of rheumatoid arthritis. *Arch Pathol Lab Med.* 59:129–50, 1955.

2. Schumacher, H.R., and Kitridou, R.C. Synovitis of recent onset: a clinico-pathologic study during the first month of disease. *Arthritis Rheum.* 15:465–85, 1972.

3. Harris, E.D., Jr. Recent insights into the pathogenesis of the proliferative lesion in rheumatoid arthritis. *Arthritis Rheum.* 19:68–72, 1976.

4. Gardner, D.L. *The Pathology of Rheumatoid Arthritis*. London: Edward Arnold Ltd., 1972.

5. Lane, J.M., and Weiss, C. Review of articular cartilage collagen research. *Arthritis Rheum.* 18:553–62, 1975.

6. Dingle, J.T. The role of lysosomal enzymes in skeletal tissues. *J Bone Joint Surg.* 55-B:87–94, 1973.

7. Kimura, H., Tateishi, H., and Ziff, M. Surface ultrastructure of rheumatoid articular cartilage. *Arthritis Rheum.* 20:1085–98, 1977.

8. Fell, H.B., and Jubb, R.W. The effect of synovial tissue on the breakdown of articular cartilage in organ culture. *Arthritis Rheum.* 20:1359–71, 1977.

9. Janis, R., and Hamerman, D. Articular cartilage changes in early arthritis. *Bull Hosp Joint Dis.* (NY) 30:136–52, 1969.

10. Barland, P., Janis, R., and Sandson, J. Immunofluorescent studies of human articular cartilage. *Ann Rheum Dis.* 25:156–63, 1966.

11. Hamerman, D. Cartilage changes in the rheumatoid joint. *Clin Orthop.* 64:91–7, 1969.

12. Ali, S.Y. The degradation of cartilage matrix by an intercellular protease. *Biochem J.* 93:611–18, 1964.

13. Sapolsky, A.I., Altman, R.D., Woessner, J.F., and Howell, D.S. The action of cathepsin D in human articular cartilage on proteoglycans. *J Clin Invest.* 52:624–33, 1973.

14. Burleigh, M.C., Barrett, A.J., and Lazarus, G.S. Cathepsin B₁: a lysosomal enzyme that degrades native collagen. *Biochem J.* 137:387–98, 1974.

15. Morrison, R.I.G., Barrett, A.J., Dingle, J.T., and Prior, D. Cathepsin B₁ and D. Action on human cartilage proteoglycans. *Biochim Biophys Acta.* 302:411–19, 1973.

16. Wood, G.C., Pryce-Jones, R.H., White, D., and Nuki, G. Chondromucoprotein-degrading neutral protease activity in rheumatoid synovial fluid. *Ann Rheum Dis.* 30:73–7, 1971.

17. Sapolsky, A.I., Howell, D.S., and Woessner, J.F. Neutral proteases and cathepsin D in human articular cartilage. *J Clin Invest.* 53:1044–53, 1974.

18. Sapolsky, A.I., Keiser, H., Howell, D.S., and Woessner, J.F., Jr. Metalloproteinases of human articular cartilage that digest cartilage proteoglycan at neutral and acid pH. *J Clin Invest.* 58:1030–41, 1976.

19. Ziff, M., Gribety, M.J., and Lospalluto, J. Effect of leukocyte and synovial membrane extracts on cartilage mucoprotein. *J Clin Invest.* 39:405–12, 1960.

20. Weissman, G., and Spilberg, I. Breakdown of cartilage protein-polysaccharide by lysosomes. *Arthritis Rheum.* 11:162–9, 1968.

21. Herman, J.H., Musgrave, D.S., and Dennis, M.V. Phytomitogen-induced, lymphokine-mediated cartilage proteoglycan degradation. *Arthritis Rheum.* 20:922–32, 1977.

22. Greenwald, R.A., Moy, W.W., and Lazarus, D. Degradation of cartilage proteoglycans and collagen by superoxide radical, abstracted. *Arthritis Rheum.* 19:799, 1976.

23. Lack, C.H. Chrondrolysis in arthritis. *J Bone Joint Surg.* 41-B:384–7, 1959.

24. Thomas, L. Reversible collapse of rabbit ears after intravenous papain, and prevention of recovery by cortisone. *J Exp Med.* 104:245–53, 1956.

25. Gross, J.I., Matthews, M.B., and Dorfman, A. Sodium chondroitin sulfate-protein complexes of cartilage. II. Metabolism. *J Biol Chem.* 235:2889–92, 1960.

26. Mankin, H.J. The structure, chemistry, and metabolism of articular cartilage. *Bull Rheum Dis.* 17:447–52, 1967.

27. Jacoby, R.K., and Jayson, M.I.V. Synthesis of glycosaminoglycan in adult human articular cartilage in organ culture from patients with rheumatoid arthritis. *Ann Rheum Dis.* 35:32–6, 1976.

28. Lowther, D. A., and Gillard, G. C. Carrageenin-induced arthritis. I. The effect of intraarticular carrageenin on the chemical composition of articular cartilage. *Arthritis Rheum.* 19:769–76, 1976.

29. Harris, E.D., Jr., and Krane, S.M. An endopeptidase from rheumatoid synovial culture. *Biochim Biophys Acta.* 258:566–76, 1972.

30. Harris, E.D., Jr. A collagenolytic system produced by primary cultures of rheumatoid nodule tissue. *J Clin Invest.* 51:2973–6, 1972.

31. Harris, E.D., Jr., and Krane, S.M. Collagenases. *N Engl J Med.* 291:557–63, 605–9, 652–61, 1974.

32. Eisen, A.Z., Bauer, E.A., and Jeffery, J.J. Human skin collagenase: the role of serum alpha-globulins in the control of activity in vivo and in vitro. *Proc Natl Acad Sci USA.* 68:248–51, 1971.

33. Kobayashi, I., and Ziff, M. Electron microscopic studies of the cartilage-pannus junction in rheumatoid arthritis. *Arthritis Rheum.* 18:475–83, 1975.

34. Woolley, D.E., Crossley, M.J., and Evanson, J.M. Collagenase at sites of cartilage erosion in the rheumatoid joint. *Arthritis Rheum.* 20:1231–9, 1977.

35. Dingle, J.T., Horsfield, P., Fell, H.B., and Barratt, M.E.J. Breakdown of proteoglycan and collagen induced in pig articular cartilage in organ culture. *Ann Rheum Dis.* 34:303–11, 1975.

36. Steffen, C. Consideration of pathogenesis of rheumatoid arthritis as collagen autoimmunity. *Z Immunitaetsforsch.* 139:219–27, 1970.

37. Cracchiolo, A., III, Michaeli, D., Goldberg, L.S., and Fudenberg, H.H. The occurrence of antibodies to collagen in synovial fluids. *Clin Immunol Immunopathol.* 3:567–74, 1975.

38. Herman, J.H., Wiltse, D.W., and Dennis, M.V. Immunopathologic significance of cartilage antigenic components in rheumatoid arthritis. *Arthritis Rheum.* 16:287–97, 1973.

39. Hollister, J.R., Liang, G., and Mannik, M. Immunologically induced acute synovitis in rabbits. *Arthritis Rheum.* 16:10–20, 1973.

40. Hollister, J.R., and Mannik, M. Antigen retention in joint tissues in antigen-induced synovitis. *Clin Exp. Immunol.* 16:615–27, 1974.

41. Hollister, J.R. Inflammatory potential of tissue-bound immune complexes. *Abstracts of the XIV International Congress of Rheumatology,* p. 97, 1977.

42. Cooke, T.D., Hurd, E.R., Jasin, H.E. et al. Identification of immunoglobulins and complement in rheumatoid articular collagenous tissues. *Arthritis Rheum.* 18:541–51, 1975.

43. Ishikawa, H., Smiley, J.D., and Ziff, M. Electron microscopic demonstration of immunoglobulin deposition in rheumatoid cartilage. *Arthritis Rheum.* 18:563–76, 1975.

44. Deshmukh, K., and Hemrick, S. Metabolic changes in rabbit articular cartilage due to inflammation. *Arthritis Rheum.* 19:199–208, 1976.

45. Bernstein, B., Forrester, D., Singsen, B. et al. Hip joint restoration in juvenile rheumatoid arthritis. *Arthritis Rheum.* 20:1099–1104, 1977.

8 HLA Antigens in Juvenile Rheumatoid Arthritis

David A. Stempel
and Andrew J. McMichael

In recent years there have been numerous reports of increased frequencies of certain HLA antigens in specific diseases, some of which are very striking.[1,2] HLA-DW3 is found in 98% of patients with celiac disease compared to 15% of controls,[3] and HLA-B27 is found in 85% to 95% of patients with ankylosing spondylitis (AS) compared to 7% of controls.[4,5] Furthermore, in populations where these antigens are rare the diseases are infrequent. In the Japanese both HLA-DW3 and celiac disease are absent[6] and HLA-B27 is very rare but is still associated with ankylosing spondylitis.[7] Other associations appear less striking but could be important because there could be etiological differences or other subgroups within the disease and because weak associations might only reflect a weak linkage disequilibrium between a disease susceptibility gene and the HLA marker gene. In this chapter the association of the HLA system with juvenile rheumatic disease is discussed in relation to the important insight that these associations shed on disease etiology.

First it is important to consider what an HLA association means. The HLA antigens are controlled by a single genetic complex on chromosome 6. A positive association must mean that either HLA antigen or a linked gene is involved in the disease process. Further, if it is a linked gene there must be linkage disequilibrium in the population between the disease susceptibility gene and the marker gene controlling HLA antigen. Linkage disequilibrium is a phenomenon in which particular alleles (alternative products) of two or more linked genetic loci occur together in the population at a greater than expected frequency. A good example is the linkage disequilibrium between HLA-A1 and B8. They are allelic products of two different HLA loci, A and B, separated by a crossover distance of 0.8% (i.e., recombination occurs between HLA A and B in 0.8% of human offspring). The gene frequency of A1 is 0.15 and of B8 is 0.12. Provided that neither allele is a recent mutation enough recombinations should have occurred between these two loci during the past several generations to allow these alleles to be treated as independent variables. The expected frequency of the haplotype A1-B8 is therefore 0.15×0.12 which is 0.02. The actual frequency is 0.07, over three times that expected, and reflects linkage disequilibrium. If B8 was a disease susceptibility gene with no recognizable antigenic marker a disease association with A1 would be seen, such that if B8 was an essential etiological factor in the disease some 50% of patients would possess A1. If there was no linkage disequilibrium, no HLA-A association would be apparent. Thus a negative HLA association does not exclude the HLA system from playing a role in the disease process and a weak association could simply reflect a weak linkage disequilibrium.

It is also important to note that all disease associations so far described are dominant associations with disease *susceptibility*. Associations with *resistance* have not been described, possibly because decreased antigen frequencies in patients are statistically much harder to prove. Nevertheless, they almost certainly exist and the mere fact that the HLA system is polymorphic and shows linkage disequilibrium implies that certain alleles and haplotypes have conferred selective survival advantages during recent human evolution.[8] Most of the diseases for which association with HLA antigens are known have unknown etiologies, probably of an autoimmune nature.

GENETIC STRUCTURE OF THE HLA AND H-2 SYSTEMS

In order to understand the possible mechanism that might explain the HLA and disease association it is necessary to consider the structure of the HLA complex and its mouse counterpart, H-2. Figure 1 shows a genetic map of the HLA complex. There are four loci, A, B, C, and D, each controlling cell surface antigens.[9] The A, B, and C antigens provoke rapid graft rejection. They are glycoproteins of 45,000 molecular weight and are associated at the cell surface with β2 microglobulin.[10] They are present on all nucleated cells. The D antigens provoke the mixed lymphocyte reaction (the proliferative response of a lymphocyte population when mixed with foreign lymphocytes).[9] On this basis the HLA D region is probably equivalent to the mouse H-2 I region which controls the expression of Ia antigens. These are smaller (33,000 molecular weight) glycoproteins expressed only on lymphocytes, macrophages, epithelial cells, and sperm.[11] They can now be detected on human lymphocytes, but although linked to HLA they have not been mapped. The A, B, C, and D antigens are all very polymorphic with multiple alleles (alternative specificities) at each locus, Figure 1, and the number of possible HLA A-B-C-D haplotypes is more than nine thousand. The complement components C2, C4 and properdin factor B (Bf) all map in the HLA complex, but their positions are uncertain.[9]

The mouse H-2 complex is similar.[12] H-2 K, and D are serologically and chemically equivalent to HLA A, B, and C. The S region controls C4. The I region controls Ia antigens and is divided into five subregions, A, B, J, E, and C.

The different map order of equivalent products does not pose great problems. The most likely explanation is that a partial chromosomal inversion occurred in one or the other species line.

Functions of the H-2 System

The relevance of this mouse H-2 system to human disease is in a considerable body of data demonstrating that H-2 products regulate immune responses.[12,13,16]

Three regulatory effects are known though the distinction between them may be somewhat artificial. First, McDevitt and coworkers showed that the immune response to certain simple antigens is quantitatively controlled by autosomal dominant immune response (Ir) genes that map in the I region of the H-2 complex.[14] These genes operate at the level of the helper T lymphocytes and probably affect T cell recognition of antigens in association with macrophages.[13] It is likely that all antigenic determinants are under this kind of control but that most complex antigens have multiple determinants so that Ir gene effects on such antigens are only seen experimentally at limiting doses.[15] Ir gene expression is not limited only to T-helper cells affecting antibody production but also to those that control generation of cytotoxic (killer) T cells[16] and the cells that proliferate in response to antigens in vitro.[15-17] Recent data suggest that as well as Ir genes regulating T-helper function there is a parallel set of H-2 linked (Is) genes relating suppressor T cell function.[18]

The second type of function in which the I region is involved is in immune cell-cell interactions. Ia antigens appear to be involved in the interactions between macrophages and T cells, suppressor T cells and B cells, and helper T cells and B cells.[11] These interactions can be mediated by soluble factors which carry I region determinants and which may show antigen specificity.[17,19] The relationship between the function of Ia antigens in cell recognition and Ir genes in antigen recognition is not clear and is the subject of intense investigation in mice.[12,13,19]

The third function controlled by the mouse H-2 complex is the killing of virus-infected cells, chemically altered cells, or cells differing

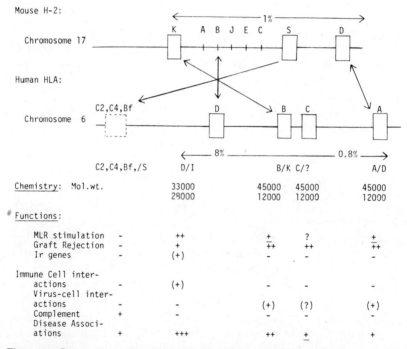

Figure 1. Structure and functions of major histocompatibility complexes of mouse (H-2) and man (HLA). Upper part shows chromosome maps for mouse H-2 and human HLA complexes. Arrows connect loci or regions that are probably equivalent. Lower part figure summarizes properties of products of each locus, shown with its HLA/H-2 designation. Functions shown in brackets, (+), are well established in mice but have not yet been conclusively demonstrated or mapped in man.

in minor histocompatibility antigens. Zinkernagel and Doherty showed that lymphocytes from lymphocytic choriomeningitis (LCM) virus-infected animals would lyse, in vitro, foreign target cells that were infected with the virus, provided that they shared H-2 K or D antigens with the killer cell.[20] This finding has now been extended for several other viruses in mice. Two explanations are possible. One is that T cells have a dual recognition system: one receptor specific for virus and the other for H-2 K and D. The other is that virus alters H-2 antigens which are then recognized as foreign by T cells: the altered self hypothesis.

Blanden et al.[21] and Nabholz and Miggiano[22] have proposed a theory whereby the H-2 system acts as a kind of receptor system for foreign viruses or proteins. These alter H-2 K or D (viruses) or Ia (proteins) which are thus recognized as foreign by T cells programmed to recognize altered self components. This immune surveillance hypothesis could also explain why such a high proportion of T cells participate in the mixed lymphocyte reaction.[23] The Ir gene effects could be explained by antigens that failed to alter particular H-2 Ia antigens. Attractive though this theory is, there is no direct evidence in its favor.

Functions of the HLA System

Data on these three kinds of function in humans are sparse. Attempts have been made to demonstrate Ir genes directly. Levine et al.[24] and Bias and Marsh[25] have population data suggesting that the immune response to grass pollen antigens is under Ir gene control.[24,25] Further, Greenberg et al.[26] and Spencer et al.[27] have population data showing that high or low responsiveness to particular antigens is associated with certain HLA types. While family studies have been less helpful study of immune cell interactions is more promising.[28,29] Taussig et al. have demonstrated that the ability of B cells to accept a mouse T cell factor specific for a peptide antigen (TGAL) is HLA-linked.[30] McMichael et al. (unpublished data) have found a suppressor T cell factor that requires HLA B and D identity between the cell producing it and the cell accepting it suggesting that this B and D region includes the functional equivalent of the mouse I region. Goulmy et al.[31] have shown that T cell cytotoxicity against the male transplantation antigen H-Y requires HLA A region identity between effector cell and target for killing to occur. A requirement for HLA B region identities has now been shown in the lymphocyte mediated lysis of influenza virus infected cells.[32]

These results suggest that the HLA complex mediates the same kind of regulating effect on the immune response as the H-2 region of the mouse. It is not possible yet to map these functions clearly; however, it is widely assumed that HLA D is equivalent to a part or the whole of the H-2 I region and that HLA A, B, and C are functionally equivalent to H-2 K and D. If these assumptions are correct the diseases most strongly associated with an HLA D antigen might be due to an Ir gene or Is gene effect. Those associated primarily with HLA A, B, or C antigen could be due to a harmful intervention between HLA and a virus. Table 1 shows those diseases in which HLA typing has been most complete, and in which a strong association with an HLA antigen has been shown.

MECHANISMS OF HLA AND DISEASE ASSOCIATION

Knowledge of the functions of the H-2 complex in the mouse thus yields clues as to possible mechanisms to explain the association of the HLA system with disease susceptibility in man.[2] Of the genes linked to the antigenic markers, Ir or Is genes are obvious candidates as they may critically affect the individual's immune response to pathogens or self components. The fact that for complex antigens Ir genes are only apparent when limiting immunizing doses are used experimentally may be relevant. The immune system of a high responder may be primed by low doses of virus proteins during subclinical infection, or the immune system may be more rapidly brought into play during an infection.

The effect of the H-2 or HLA polymorphism on immunocyte interactions has yet to be studied. However, subtle variations in immune responses might occur with different alleles or haplotypes.

Virus interaction with HLA A, B, and C antigens, which is predicted from mouse experiments, could explain the greater associations found with these antigens in certain diseases, (e.g., B27 with ankylosing spondylitis). Again, if the various allelic cell-surface products each interacted with varying efficiency with different viruses, there might be marked variation in susceptibility to viral diseases with different HLA types. Intracellular bacteria and parasites could have similar effects.

Genetic variation in the complement components could also explain some HLA and disease associations. C2 deficiency associated with the HLA haplotype A10-BW18-DW2 has been found and some of these individuals have a lupuslike disease.[33] While electrophoretic variants of C2, C4, and Bf have been described little is known of functional

Table 1
Principal locus associations for 15 diseases

	Locus A	Locus B	Locus C	Locus D	
Hemochromatosis	A3	Ankylosing spondylitis	B27	Psoriasis	C7	Multiple sclerosis	DW3
Congenital Heart	A2	Reiter's disease	B27			Celiac disease	DW3
disease						Graves' disease	DW3
						Juvenile-onset diabetes	DW3
						Addison's disease	DW3
						Sjogren's syndrome	DW3
						Chronic active	DW3
						hepatitis	
						Myasthenia gravis	DW3
						Rheumatoid arthritis	DW4
						Vogt-Harada's disease	LD AH
						Psoriasis	LD MA

Each disease is listed under the locus with which it shows the strongest association. The relevant antigen is also shown. For these diseases associations have been sought with antigens at the A, B, C, and D loci, except for patients with hemochromatosis and congenital heart disease where D typing has not been done. See References 1 and 2.

variability. However, since the complement system mediates immune injury it is clear that variability here could play a role in disease susceptibility.

Other possible mechanisms involve the HLA gene products themselves. These are less likely explanations except in instances where the association approaches 100%. It is possible that certain pathogens could mimic an HLA antigen and thereby escape immune recognition in individuals with that antigen, however, no evidence has yet been presented in support of this hypothesis. HLA antigens could facilitate virus replication by, for instance, their incorporation in the virus coat as described in the mouse by Bubbers and Lilly for the Friend leukemia virus and H-2 D^b.[34] A particular HLA antigen could also act as a pathogen or toxin receptor although there is no experimental evidence in favor of this hypothesis.

Finally, linked genes that are not involved in immune responses should be considered as candidates. Most diseases shown to be associated with HLA antigens had previously been thought to have an immune component in their etiology. However, diseases such as psoriasis, hemochromatosis, and congenital heart defects do not normally have associated immunologic abnormalities. It is of interest therefore, that the H-2 system in the mouse has been shown to control the level of cyclic AMP in the liver[35] and of serum testosterone,[36] findings which may indicate a more generalized cell surface receptor role for these molecules. It has been suggested that the HLA or H-2 system is part of a larger genetic complex controlling cell-cell recognitions and that the part controlling immune cell recognition has been discovered first because experimental techniques are available.[8] If this is correct the possible mechanisms for disease association become multitudinous. However, there is as yet no evidence to suggest that this hypothesis is correct and for the present, genetic variability in immune function seems to be the most likely general explanation for the HLA and disease associations.

Associations with Juvenile Rheumatoid Arthritis (JRA)

The study of the HLA antigens and rheumatic diseases in children has been rewarding. HLA-B27 is strongly associated in children, as in adults, with ankylosing spondylitis (AS).[4,5] Prevalence of HLA-B27 in Reiter's syndrome,[37] reactive arthropathy,[38] acute anterior uveitis,[39] and inflammatory bowel disease with sacroiliitis[40] is increased. Studies of association of D antigens to JRA appear promising.[41-43]

The association of HLA-B27 and AS in adults is well established. Schlosstein et al. described 40 patients with AS, 88% of whom had HLA-B27.[5] They also studied patients with rheumatoid arthritis and gout and could find no association between HLA-B27 or the 23 other antigens tested. Brewerton et al. found B27 in 95% of 75 patients with AS as well as in 52% of their asymptomatic first degree relatives which indicates that disease activity or its treatment are not responsible for the antigen's presence.[4] Although the prevalence of HLA-B27 antigen is rare in the Japanese, it is common among those with AS (67%).[7]

In the Haida Indians of North America the frequency of HLA-B27 is 50%, 20% of whom have AS. Gene frequency of B27 in this population and the occurrence of AS correlate well. Six of 17 patients studied in this tribe with AS are homozygous or homozygous state. In other closed American Indian populations with increased prevalence of B27, the association still exists but the expression of clinical disease is not as marked.[44]

The association of B27 and AS is significant in that it may be of help in the early diagnosis of AS. Further epidemiological study by Calin and Fries suggests that the actual incidence of AS is closer to 20% of B27-positive individuals, and that the male-female ratio is 1:1.[45] They believe an increased awareness of the correlation between B27 and AS would lead to more effective therapy. This genetic marker hopefully will lead to a better understanding of the pathogenesis of the disease. The association of Reiter's syndrome, post-*Shigella* arthritis and *Yersinia* arthritis with B27 is intriguing and lends evidence to the belief that the human analog of the mouse immune response gene exists.

Brewerton et al. speculated on the presence of B27 antigen in patients with JRA.[4] Noting that adolescent boys with lower limb arthropathy frequently develop AS, they speculated that B27 might be found in this population and aid in early diagnosis of AS. Subsequent investigations by several laboratories have resulted in conflicting reports. The initial study by Rachelefsky et al. found B27 in 42% of patients with JRA.[46] Those with the B27 antigen had early onset, negative rheumatoid factor, and no difference in sex distribution. A large number of reports confirming and denying these data followed. Gibson et al.[47] and Mitsiu et al.,[48] the latter in a study of Japanese with JRA, were unable to show an association between JRA and B27 after those patients with AS or sacroiliitis were excluded from the study. Gibson found that seven of 12 children with JRA and tenosynovitis were positive for HLA-B27.

Schaller et al. found a 26% prevalence of B27 among 112 patients with JRA.[49] After dividing the study population into seven clinical groups based on type of onset, rheumatoid factor (RF), chronic iridocyclitis, and sex, only two subpopulations had a statistically increased frequency of B27: those with AS and boys with pauciarticular disease. Sacroiliitis and acute iridocyclitis were found in this group. Onset in these patients was later in childhood, involved the lower extremities, and was associated with both a negative RF test and antinuclear antibody. Schaller also found increased frequency of A2 and BW15 in polyarticular RF-negative populations. Veys et al. confirmed this association again, noting that when one studies the evolution of JRA a distinct subpopulation exists with a clinical picture of AS or of developing AS.[50] B27, therefore, serves as a marker in patients with JRA by identifying a group of children presenting with lower limb arthropathy who may go on to develop AS or at least sacroiliitis. It also reinforces the evidence that JRA is in fact several diseases with different clinical manifestations.

Brewerton et al. noted a 55% incidence of HLA-B27 in 50 adults with acute anterior uveitis.[39] A significant number of those had AS or some form of spondylitis. Studies of children have noted an association of B27 with acute anterior uveitis, but not with chronic iridocyclitis. Ohno et al. studied 43 children with the latter disease and found no correlation with the B27 antigen or the other HLA antigens.[51] He studied 23 patients with JRA and chronic iridocyclitis of whom 22 had monoarticular or pauciarticular disease and none had acute anterior uveitis. A high proportion of the children studied with chronic uveitis had positive antinuclear antibodies.

Initial studies into the immunogenetics of rheumatic diseases were limited to serologically defined loci. The associations of DW3 with diseases that produce organ-specific autoantibodies such as Graves' disease, Addison's disease, and juvenile diabetes mellitus have led researchers to study this locus in relation to rheumatic disease.[2] Further interest in studying the D locus is spurred by the possibility that it is the human correlate to the mouse I region. Two studies in adults showed a significant correlation between DW4 and rheumatoid arthritis. Stastny reported that 31 of 43 patients with rheumatoid arthritis failed to respond to antigen R (later found to correlate with DW4); another report showed a frequency of DW4 of 36% (control 13%) with an associated increase in CW3 of 35% (control 17%).[41,52] These two antigens are thought to be in linkage disequilibrium.

Gershwin et al., in a report of 46 patients with JRA found a 64% incidence of DW3 in children (control 15%) with polyarticular and systemic disease.[42] They did not find an increased incidence of B8 as one might expect because of the linkage disequilibrium with DW3. Stastny et al. reported no increased prevalence of DW3 or DW4 in 110 children with JRA.[43] They studied a new determinant, LD-TMo, noting its incidence in 33% of 58 children with pauciarticular JRA and none of 35 normal controls. We have studied 41 children with JRA and have also been unable to confirm Gershwin's finding (D.A. Stempel, A.J. McMichael, and J.J. Miller, III, unpublished data). Out of 17 children with polyarticular disease, and five with systemic onset, only one had DW3. We found a 14% incidence (control 15%) of DW4 in those with polyarticular disease. Other subpopulation groups in our study are too limited at present to make a statement. As the B cell alloantisera become better defined more complete studies can be performed.

Reports of associations between other collagen vascular disease with HLA antigens have been made. Dermatomyositis appears to be associated with A1 and B8, and therefore presumably to DW3.[53] Sjogren's syndrome has been associated with antigen B8 in 59% and with DW3 in 69% of patients studied.[54] The stronger association with DW3 demonstrates that the susceptibility gene is closer to the D locus.

CONCLUSION

The HLA associations with JRA are weak if one defines it as one disease. However, when one considers HLA-B27–positive JRA patients a strong clinical correlation is made with sacroiliitis and potential to develop AS. As serological markers are found which are controlled by genes that map closer to the disease susceptibility genes, much stronger associations should become apparent. The current work in progress on defining the human Ia antigens and their genetic loci will prove of great interest. By analogy with the mouse, these antigens should be very closely related to immune response genes which are presently the best candidates for disease susceptibility genes. It is anticipated, therefore, that typing for Ia antigens in many diseases will reveal associations as striking as those already found for celiac disease and multiple sclerosis.[55] The prospects are good that several syndromes now grouped as JRA may become distinct when studied, which will not only allow identification of susceptible individuals but will open the way to better understanding of the disease process.

REFERENCES

1. Moller, G., editor. HLA and disease. *Transplant Rev.* 22, 1975.

2. McMichael, A.H., and McDevitt, H.O. The association between HLA antigens and disease. *Progress in Medical Genetics.* (In press)

3. Kuening, J.J., Pena, A.S., van Leeuwen, A. et al. HLA-DW3 associated with coeliac disease. *Lancet.* 1:506–7, 1976.

4. Brewerton, D.A., Caffrey, M., Hart, F.D. et al. Ankylosing spondylitis and HL-A27. *Lancet.* 1:904–7, 1973.

104

5. Schlosstein, L., Terasaki, P.I., Bluestone, R., and Pearson, C.M. High association of an HL-A antigen, W27, with ankylosing spondylitis. *N Engl J Med*. 288:704–6, 1973.

6. Sasazuki, T., McMichael, A.J., Payne, R., and McDevitt, H.O. HLA haplotype differences between Japanese and Caucasians. *Tissue Antigens*. (In press)

7. Sonozaki, H., Seki, H., Chang, S. et al. Human lymphocyte antigen HL-A27, in Japanese patients with ankylosing spondylitis. *Tissue Antigens*. 5:131–6, 1975.

8. Bodmer, W.F. Evolutionary significance of the HL-A system. *Nature*. 237:139–45, 1972.

9. Kissmey-Nielssen, F., editor. *Histocompatibility Testing*. Copenhagen: Munksgaard, 1975.

10. Crumpton, M.J., and Snary, D. Isolation and characterization of human histocompatibility (HLA) antigens. *Current Topics in Immunochemistry*. (In press)

11. Hämmerling, G.J., Mauve, G., Goldberg, E., and McDevitt, H.O. Tissue distribution of Ia antigens: Ia on spermatozoa, macrophages and epidermal cells. *Immunogenetics*. 1:428–37, 1975.

12. Klein, J. *Biology of the Mouse Histocompatibility-2 Complex*. New York: Springer-Verlag, 1975.

13. Katz, D.H., and Benacerraf, B., editors. *The Role of the Histocompatibility Gene Complex in the Immune Response*. New York: Academic Press, 1974.

14. Benacerraf, B., and McDevitt, H.O. Histocompatibility-linked immune response genes. *Science*. 175:273–9, 1972.

15. Vaz, N.M., Phillips-Quagliata, J.M., Levine, B.B., and Vaz, E.M. H-2 linked genetic control of immune responsiveness of ovalbumin and ovomucoid. *J Exp Med*. 134:1335–48, 1971.

16. Schmitt-Verhulst, A., and Schearer, G.M. Bifunctional major histocompatibility-linked genetic regulation of cell-mediated lympholysis to trinitrophenyl-modified autologous lymphocytes. *J Exp Med*. 142:914–27, 1975.

17. Lonai, P., and McDevitt, H.O. Genetic control of the immune response. In vitro stimulation of lymphocytes by (T, G)-A–L, (H, G)-A–L and (Phe, G)-A–L. *J Exp Med*. 140:977–94, 1974.

18. Kapp, J.A., Pierce, C.W., Schlossman, S., and Benacerraf, B. Genetic control of immune responses in vitro. V. Stimulation of suppressor T cells in nonresponder mice by the terpolymer L-glutamic acid[60]-L–alanine[30]-L–tyrosin[10] (GAT). *J Exp Med*. 140:648–59, 1974.

19. Herzenberg, L., Sercarz, E., and Fox, C.F., editors. *Proceedings of the 1977 ICN-UCLA Symposium. Regulation of the immune response*. (In press)

20. Zinkernagel, R.M., and Doherty, P.C. Immunological surveillance against altered self components by sensitized T-lymphocytes in lymphocytic choriomeningitis. *Nature*. 251:547–8, 1974.

21. Blanden, R.V., Hapel, A.J., and Jackson, D.C. Speculation: mode of action of Ir genes and the nature of T cell receptors for antigens. *Immunochemistry*. 13:179–91, 1976.

22. Nabholz, M., and Miggiano, V. The Biological Significance of the Mixed Leukocyte Reaction in B and T Cells. Edited by F. Loor. In *Immune Recognition*. London: Wiley and Sons, Int. Publ. Co., 1977.

23. Kreth, H.W., and Williamson, A.R. Cell surveillance model for lymphocyte cooperation. *Nature*. 234:454–6, 1971.

24. Levine, B.B., Stember, R.H., and Fotino, M. Ragweed hayfever: genetic control and linkage to HLA haplotypes. *Science*. 178:1201–3, 1972.

25. Bias, W.B., and Marsh, D.G. HL-A linked antigen E immune response genes: an unproved hypothesis. *Science*. 188:375–7, 1975.

26. Greenberg, L.J., Gray, E.D., and Unis, E.J. Association of HL-A5 and immune responsiveness in vitro to streptococcal antigens. *J Exp Med*. 141:935–43, 1975.

27. Spencer, M.J., Cherry, J.O., and Terasaki, P.I. HL-A antigens and antibody response after Influenza A vaccination. Decreased response associated with HL-A type W16. *N Engl J Med*. 294:13–16, 1976.

28. McMichael, A.J., Sasazuki, T., and McDevitt, H.O. The immune response to diphtheria toxoid in humans. *Transplant Proc*. 9 (suppl 1):191–4, 1977.

29. Black, P.L., Marsh, D.G., Jarrett, E. et al. Family study of association between HLA and specific immune responses to highly purified pollen allergens. *Immunogenetics*. 3:349–68, 1976.

30. Taussig, M., Luzatti, A., and Cepellini, R. Paper presented at the First International Congress of HLA and Disease, Paris, 1976.

31. Gaulmy, E., Termijtelen, A., Bradley, B.A., and van Rood, J.J. Y-antigen killing by T cells of women is restricted by HLA. *Nature*. 266:544–6, 1977.

32. McMichael, A.J., Ting, A., Zweerink, H.J., and Askonas, B.A. HLA restriction of cell mediated-lysis of influenza virus-infected human cells. *Nature*. 270:524–6, 1977.

33. Stern, R., Fu, S.M., Fotino, M. et al. Hereditary C2 deficiency: association with skin lesions resembling the discoid lesions of systemic lupus erythematosus. *Arthritis Rheum*. 19:517–22, 1976.

34. Bubbers, J.E., and Lilly, F. Selective incorporation of H-2 antigenic determinants into Friend virus particles. *Nature*. 266:458–9, 1977.

35. Meruelo, D., and Edidin, M. Association of mouse liver adenine 3′,5′-cyclic monophosphate (cyclic AMP) levels with histocompatibility-2 genotype. *Proc Natl Acad Sci*. 72:2644–8, 1975.

36. Ivani, P., Gregorova, S., and Mickova, M. Genetic differences in thymus, lymph node, testis, and vesicular gland weights among inbred mouse strains. Association with histocompatibility (2) system. *Folia Biol*. (Prague) 19:81, 1972.

37. Brewerton, D.A., Nicholls, A., Oates, J.K. et al. Reiter's disease and HL-A27. *Lancet*. 2:996–8, 1973.

38. Aho, K., Ahvonen, P., Alkio, P. et al. HL-A27 in reactive arthritis following infection. *Ann Rheum Dis*. 34 (suppl):29–30, 1975.

39. Brewerton, D.A., Nicholls, A., Caffrey, M. et al. Acute anterior uveitis and HL-A27. *Lancet*. 2:994–6, 1973.

40. Morris, R.I., Metzger, A.L., Bluestone, R., and Terasaki, P.I. HLA-W27: a useful discriminator in the arthropathies of inflammatory bowel disease. *N Engl J Med*. 290:1117–19, 1974.

41. Stastny, P. Mixed lymphocyte cultures in rheumatoid arthritis. *J Clin Invest*. 57:1148–57, 1976.

42. Gershwin, M.E., Opelz, G., Terasaki, P.I. et al. HLA-D and Ia-type alloantigens in juvenile rheumatoid arthritis, abstracted. *Clin Research*. 25:118, 1977.

43. Stastny, P., and Fink, C.S. Different associations of HLA-D locus antigens with adult and juvenile rheumatoid arthritis, abstracted. Program of the XIV International Congress of Rheumatology. p. 181, 1977.

44. Gofton, J.P., Chalmers, A., Price, G.E., and Reeve, C.E. HL-A27 and ankylosing spondylitis in B.C. Indians. *J Rheumatol.* 2:314–18, 1975.

45. Calin, A., and Fries, J.F. Striking prevalence of ankylosing spondylitis in "healthy" W27 positive males and females. A controlled study. *N Engl J Med.* 293:835–9, 1975.

46. Rachelefsky, G.S., Terasaki, P.I., Katz, R., and Stiehm, E.R. Increased prevalence of W27 in juvenile rheumatoid arthritis. *N Engl J Med.* 290:892–3, 1974.

47. Gibson, D.J., Carpenter, C.B., Stillman, J.S., and Schur, P.H. Reexamination of histocompatibility antigens found in patients with juvenile rheumatoid arthritis. *N Engl J Med.* 293:636–8, 1975.

48. Mitsui, H., Juni, T., Sonozaki, H. et al. Distribution of HLA-B27 in patients with juvenile rheumatoid arthritis. *Ann Rheum Dis.* 36:86–7, 1977.

49. Schaller, J.G., Ochs, H.D., Thomas, E.D. et al. Histocompatibility antigens in childhood-onset arthritis. *J Pediatr.* 88:926–30, 1976.

50. Veys, E.M., Coigne, E., Mielants, H., and Verbrugten, G. HLA and juvenile chronic polyarthritis. *J Rheumatol.* 4 (suppl 3):74–7, 1977.

51. Ohno, S., Char, D.H., Kimura, S.J., and O'Connor, G.R. HLA antigens and antinuclear antibody titres in juvenile chronic iridocyclitis. *Br J Ophthalmol.* 61:59–61, 1977.

52. McMichael, A.J., Sasazuki, T., McDevitt, H.O., and Payne, R.O. Increased frequency of HLA-CW3 and HLA-DW4 in rheumatoid arthritis. *Arthritis Rheum.* 20:1037–42, 1977.

53. Cannon, R.A., Jonasson, O., and Pachman, L.M. HLA phenotypes in childhood dermatomyositis. *Arthritis Rheum.* 20 (suppl):499, 1977.

54. Hinzova, E., Ivanyi, D., Sula, K. et al. HLA-DW3 in Sjogren's syndrome. *Tissue Antigens.* 9:8–10, 1977.

55. Winchester, R.J., Ebers, G., Fu, S.M. et al. B-cell alloantigen Ag 7a in multiple sclerosis. *Lancet* 2:814, 1975.

SECTION II

Clinical Aspects

9 Still's Disease: Systemic Juvenile Rheumatoid Arthritis

Linda J. Gorin

PRESENTATION

General

One of the more dramatic, sometimes frightening, often perplexing presentations of juvenile rheumatoid arthritis (JRA) is the systemic form. This mode of onset, referred to in the past as "Still's disease" or "acute febrile onset," occurs in 20% to 44% of reported series.[1-6] Arthritis may be absent initially and for as long as four months to nine years after onset of fever in as many as 50% of systemic patients.[7-10] During this delay these children are frequently subjected to intensive and invasive workups for infection, malignancy, and obscure causes of fevers of unknown origin. Even with a correct diagnosis in hand physicians faced with a pale, hyperpyrexic, often wasted and pained child may find it difficult to refrain from using aggressive steroid therapy to obtain rapid resolution. Indeed, to some extent this anxiousness is justified since the systemic onset group seems to include the majority of arthritis patients at risk of death or severe complications from

109

infection, pericarditis, myocarditis, or hepatic sensitivity to drug therapy (in particular, salicylates).[8,11-13]

Age at onset is under five years for most and so these are the younger patients described in arthritis populations. The youngest reported case, was six weeks and the median age is four to five years.[3-5,9,10] Male patients equal or slightly outnumber females in contrast to other JRA onset types.

Fever

Daily or twice-daily fevers of 103°F or greater with rapid return to normal or subnormal temperature is characteristic of this subset of patients. This fever is more hectic than that of acute rheumatic fever (ARF), having higher peaks and more dramatic variations often occurring in late afternoon or evening. The fever may be preceded by shaking and chills and may be accompanied by an evanescent "rheumatoid" rash. Although sometimes significant immobilizing arthralgia may be present during febrile episodes many children without objective arthritis appear well and comfortable between fever spikes. A few become debilitated by the recurrent fever.

Large therapeutic doses of aspirin (100 mg/kg/day) can control this fever pattern. The more rapid response of fever to salicylates in ARF (24 to 48 hours) is often cited as a differential point in distinguishing ARF and JRA. Systemic JRA fever is more often slow to respond to therapy, although there are patients whose fevers prove sensitive to salicylates and some ARF patients defervesce sluggishly. Rarely the febrile component is so debilitating and resistant to salicylate therapy that steroids may be used over the short term to control this symptom. However, permanent morbidity from the extraarticular manifestations is not seen and their natural course rarely lasts more than six months.[1,14] These facts need be weighed against the recognized risks introduced by the use of steroids.

Rash

A characteristic fleeting, occasionally pruritic rash which often accompanies febrile episodes is a helpful diagnostic clue particularly in febrile patients without arthritis. Pale erythematous macules about two to 10 mm in diameter appear on the trunk and proximal extremities and less commonly on the face and distal extremities (including the palms and soles). Individual lesions tend to change location and the larger ones may be intensified by or elicited by heat, embarrassment, or rubbing or scratching the skin. The latter phenomenon is known as an isomorphic response or Koebner phenomenon. Rash is present in 40% to 95% of systemic onset patients and may be recurrent for months or years even in the absence of other signs of disease activity.[1,2,10,15]

Arthralgia

The patients usually have significant arthralgia, if not arthritis, resulting in a characteristic posture of anxious guarded flexion of all extremities. Lingering in bed or crankiness when dressing may be a reflection of morning stiffness in the young child. Cervical spine involvement is seen in 50% to 65% of patients and results in use of the entire torso in turning so that the patient is described as "moving like a robot."[2,16]

Myalgia

Myalgia may be striking, particularly at the height of fever. However, CPK values, when reported, have not been remarkable in patients not yet on salicylates.[17]

Hepatomegaly

Liver enlargement sometimes as massive as 10 cm below the costal margin occurs in systemic JRA, usually at the onset of disease.[18] Histologically, before salicylate therapy, biopsies have shown only hyperplasia of Kupffer cells and nonspecific periportal collections of inflammatory cells, primarily small lymphocytes or mononuclear cells.[18] Hepatocellular necrosis has not been described, nor have the reported abnormalities of liver function been dramatic. SGOT values have ranged from two to eight times normal, with SGPT values usually minimally elevated (although one patient described was 20 times normal).[17,18] Bilirubin changes have been unimpressive.

There have been several reports of hepatotoxicity of varying magnitude associated with aspirin therapy in these patients.[19,26] Some writers have raised serious questions about the ability of these seemingly mildly disturbed livers to withstand insults, i.e. aspirin or viruses, which would be minor under other circumstances.[13,15,25,26] Particularly unnerving is the report of Goel and Shanks of three hepatic deaths among their nine fatalities which the authors believed to be unrelated to aspirin therapy.[8] There are 15 hepatic deaths cited in the literature and all were patients with the systemic form of disease.[13] The importance of drug-induced liver abnormalities in this form of JRA may not yet be recognized and there may be a small number of systemic patients with a fulminant hepatic component to their disease.

Splenomegaly

The spleen may also be enlarged but is rarely palpated more than three to four cm below the costal margin. If massive enlargement is present the possibility of infection or amyloidosis should be considered. Both hepatic or splenic enlargement may be part of a diffuse hyperplasia of the reticuloendothelial system which may include mesenteric lymph nodes. All of these may contribute to the increased abdominal girth observed in patients. Serous peritonitis has also been invoked as a cause of abdominal distention in patients.[27] Abdominal pain, sometimes severe enough to lead to laparotomy, occurs in as many as 40% of patients and has been variably attributed to hepatomegaly, mesenteric adenitis, or serous peritonitis.

Lymphadenopathy

Striking generalized enlargement of lymph nodes particularly in the axilla and groin occurs in 50% to 85% of the febrile onset group with individual nodes as much as 5 cm in diameter.[1,3,14] Enlarged nodes are characteristically well circumscribed, freely movable, firm, and nontender. Their presence may be perceived as uncomfortable by the child. Striking lymphadenopathy, especially in combination with hepatosplenomegaly, may suggest lymphoma or other systemic malignancy. Marked follicular lymphoid hyperplasia has been observed and the nodes may histologically simulate lymphoma.[28,29]

Pleuritis

Part of the general serositis which occurs in this presentation is pleuritis, usually asymptomatic.[14] It has been diagnosed by x-ray in as many as one-third of patients. Parenchymal lung disease is generally not encountered.

Pericarditis

Pericarditis is the most common manifestation of polyserositis and is usually benign. Affected children generally do not complain of dyspnea or precordial pain and a friction rub is likely to be evanescent or absent.

Evidences for pericarditis are tachycardia with a normal P-R interval and abnormalities of EKG, radiographs, or echocardiography (see Chapter 13). The pericardial effusion is rarely sufficient to cause significant impairment of cardiac output or actual tamponade.[27,30] Constrictive pericarditis has not been described as a late sequelae in these patients.

Myocarditis

Myocarditis, evidenced by heart failure without pericarditis, endocarditis or hypertension has been observed and cited in three published series as the cause of death in nine out of 81 patients dying with JRA.[7,12,14,31,32] (See discussion in Chapter 13.)

Iridocyclitis

Although rare, iridocyclitis may occur in this subset of patients.[8,33,34]

Central Nervous System

Primary involvement of the central nervous system (CNS) has been inferred in patients with increased irritability, drowsiness, or meningismus. Cerebrospinal fluids have been normal but reported EEG abnormalities in patients taking no medication consist of slowing and asymmetrical focal changes.[15,35-37] Underlying CNS vasculitis or a "toxic encephalopathic" response similar to that seen in scarlet fever has been suggested but not documented to explain these findings.

Laboratory Findings

As with other presenting forms, systemic disease is not associated with any specific laboratory abnormality although some trends have been noted. Patients with acute febrile onset tend to have the most marked neutrophilic leucocytosis (20,000–80,000/mm³), thrombocytosis (sometimes as high as 1×10^6/mm³), and more pronounced anemia (hematocrit less than 28%).[3,6,14] Standard tests for rheumatoid factor and antinuclear antibody are rarely positive in patients with systemic disease.[14,38] The ESR is usually elevated. Serum protein electrophoresis may reveal elevated levels of alpha-2 and gamma globulins. Urinalysis may on occasion show slight proteinuria secondary to fever but is usually normal.

DIFFERENTIAL DIAGNOSIS

The diagnosis of systemic JRA may involve exclusion of infectious or other rheumatic diseases, particularly in the absence of arthritis. The diagnosis is most often a clinical one, but the laboratory is helpful in excluding other diseases which can mimic aspects of this illness.

Infection

Infectious causes for fever must be looked for with appropriate blood and urine cultures. Acute and convalescent sera for viral titers, as well as correct specimens for viral culture should be obtained. A Mono-Spot test is sometimes valuable to rule out infectious mononucleosis which can present with fever, rash, and polyarthritis.[39]

Malignancy

In pursuit of the etiology of a fever of unknown origin occult malignancy must be considered. This possibility is most pressing when the patient is a febrile, wasting, anemic child with dramatic lymphadenopathy and hepatosplenomegaly. Arthritis may accompany or precede the diagnosis of leukemia or lymphoma.[40,41] Usually, affected joints due to neoplasm are markedly painful out of proportion to the objective changes seen. Purpura and easy bruising are often a presenting finding in leukemia but are not seen in untreated juvenile rheumatoid arthritis. However, keep in mind that aspirin may cause excessive bruising, but that the platelet count will be normal. Thrombocytopenia, or an extremely poor response to salicylates or other antirheumatic therapy lend additional support to the consideration of malignancy. Because leukemia or lymphoma may mimic JRA for months or years, bone marrow examination is often indicated in the initial or early workup of febrile onset JRA.

Acute Rheumatic Fever

Although high antistreptolysin titers have been reported with JRA, other streptococcal antibodies have not been described as raised.[42,43] The fever of ARF does not display the dramatic wide swings of 4° to 5°C often seen with systemic JRA. Erythema marginatum is an angry, red, serpiginous rash which does not involve the face, palms or soles, and is not as quickly fleeting as the classic JRA rash.

Endocarditis is part of the pancarditis of ARF but has not been described in JRA. Pericarditis as an isolated cardiac problem is not encountered in ARF.

Involved joints in ARF are more exquisitely tender to light touch than the guarded joints of JRA, and specific joints change within hours or days. The total duration of ARF arthritis is rarely more than five weeks.[9]

Systemic Lupus Erythematosus

Most systemic JRA patients present as under four or five years of age at onset, an extremely rare occurrence for SLE.[44] Other important distinctions would be the presence of sizable proteinuria, evidence of nephritis, or hypertension, all markers of renal involvement in systemic lupus but not JRA. Malar rash and significant alopecia are helpful support for the diagnosis of SLE. The absence of positive ANAs virtually excludes SLE. They are found in JRA but are in low titer and are particularly rare among acute febrile-onset patients. Reported positive anti-DNA levels are generally low with significant titers in only 1% to 3% of JRA patients.[42] Serum complement levels are normal or somewhat elevated in JRA, as opposed to reduced values in SLE. The marked leucocytosis so characteristic of systemic JRA is absent in SLE patients who are often leucopenic. While occasionally a Coombs-positive anemia occurs in rheumatoid arthritis, it is not strongly positive, and is usually insufficient to account for the degree of anemia seen.

Table 1
Prognosis of Systemic JRA

Author	Number of Patients	Repeated Episodes of Systemic Disease	Developed Chronic Polyarthritis	Number in Disability Class III or IV*	Number Developing Hip Disease	Death among Patients with Systemic JRA/ Total Deaths of JRA Patients
Schaller[1]	22	11	21	7	—	—
Calabro[10]	40	10	8	2	—	—
Fink[4]	35	—	29	—	17	—
Goel & Shanks[8]	44	—	22	—	—	8/9
Stillman[2]	—	—	—	27%	—	—
Bernstein[12]	—	—	—	—	—	13/14

*Steinbrocker classification
Superscripts indicate references.

Serum Sickness or Hypersensitivity Angiitis

These may present with intermittent fever and vague rashes. A carefully taken history seeking an inciting agent may be helpful.

The "joint swelling" seen in these patients is often more periarticular rather than true intraarticular pathology and particularly involves the dorsum of the hands or feet. Acute glomerulonephritis occurs with acute allergic reactions but not with JRA. Striking leucocytosis or elevated sedimentation rates are unusual; but there may be a transient drop in serum CH50 in the early stages.

Other vasculitic disorders may be part of the differential alternatives but soon declare themselves. A diagnostic purpuric rash involving lower limbs and buttocks in combination with glomerulonephritis help define Schoenlein-Henoch purpura.[45] Polyarteritis nodosum displays early renal manifestations, hypertension, or coronary artery involvement, with diagnosis confirmed by skin-muscle or renal biopsy.

NATURAL HISTORY

Patients with acute febrile onset, although initially very ill, have generally been felt to have a good outlook, with systemic manifestations usually not present for more than six to nine consecutive months.[14,29] Calabro observed a 75% remission rate among these children.[10] Although many of them will follow a polycyclic course, or remit, the group also includes a high proportion of children who suffer a chronic polyarthritis with resulting disability. (Table 1.) Growth retardation is greater among systemic onset patients when compared to the two other onset modes even in the absence of steroid therapy.[46,47] Most disturbing is the seeming predominance of younger patients whose age offers a greater period of time for illness to evolve, and the increased incidence of systemic patients among the deaths reported for the JRA population in the USA.[8,11,12] The age of death reported from series outside United States is somewhat older and is associated with amyloid and its sequelae,[32] a complication rarely seen in this country.

REFERENCES

1. Schaller, J.G. Juvenile rheumatoid arthritis. Series 1. *Arthritis Rheum.* 20 (suppl):165–70, 1977.

2. Stillman, J.S., and Barry, P.E. Juvenile rheumatoid arthritis. Series 2. *Arthritis Rheum.* 20 (suppl):171–5, 1977.

118

3. Ansell, B.M. Juvenile chronic polyarthritis. Series 3. *Arthritis Rheum.* 20 (suppl):176–80, 1977.

4. Fink, C.W. Patients with JRA: a clinical study. *Arthritis Rheum.* 20 (suppl):183–4, 1977.

5. Hanson, V., Kornreich, H., Bernstein, B. et al. Three subtypes of juvenile rheumatoid arthritis. Correlations of age at onset, sex and serologic factors. *Arthritis Rheum.* 20 (suppl):184–6, 1977.

6. Levinson, J.E., Balz, G.P., and Hess, E.V. Report of studies on juvenile arthritis. *Arthritis Rheum.* 20 (suppl):189–90, 1977.

7. Calabro, J.J., Burnstein, S.L., and Staley, H.L. JRA posing as fever of unknown origin. *Arthritis Rheum.* 20 (suppl):178–80, 1977.

8. Goel, K.M., and Shanks, R.A. Followup study of 100 cases of juvenile rheumatoid arthritis. *Ann Rheum Dis.* 33:25–31, 1974.

9. Brewer, E.J., Jr. Manifestations of disease. Edited by E.J. Brewer, Jr. In *Juvenile Rheumatoid Arthritis.* Philadelphia: W.B. Saunders Co., 1970, pp. 1–47.

10. Calabro, J.J., Halgerson, W.B., Sonpal, G.M., and Khoury, M.I. Juvenile rheumatoid arthritis: a general review and report of 100 patients observed for 15 years. *Semin Arthritis Rheum.* 5:257–98, 1976.

11. Baum, J., and Gutowska, G. Death in juvenile rheumatoid arthritis. *Arthritis Rheum.* 20 (suppl):253–5, 1977.

12. Bernstein, B. Death in juvenile rheumatoid arthritis. *Arthritis Rheum.* 20 (suppl):256–7, 1977.

13. Boone, J.E. Hepatic disease and mortality in juvenile rheumatoid arthritis. *Arthritis Rheum.* 20 (suppl):257–8, 1977.

14. Schaller, J., and Wedgwood, R.J. Juvenile rheumatoid arthritis: a review. *Pediatrics.* 50:940–52, 1977.

15. Calabro, J.J. Other extra-articular manifestations of juvenile rheumatoid arthritis. *Arthritis Rheum.* 20 (suppl):237–40, 1977.

16. Bywaters, E.G. Still's disease in the adult. *Ann Rheum Dis.* 30:121–33, 1971.

17. Rachelefsky, G.S., Kar, N.C., Coulson, A. et al. Serum enzyme abnormalities in juvenile rheumatoid arthritis. *Pediatrics.* 58:730–6, 1976.

18. Schaller, J.G., Beckwith, B., and Wedgwood, R.J. Hepatic involvement in juvenile rheumatoid arthritis. *J Pediatr.* 77:203–9, 1970.

19. Kornreich, H., Malouf, N.W., and Hanson, V. Acute hepatic dysfunction in JRA. *J Pediatr.* 79:27–35, 1971.

20. Rich, R.R., and Johnson, J.S. Salicylate hepatotoxicity in patients with JRA. *Arthritis Rheum.* 16:1–9, 1973.

21. Athreya, B.H., Gorske, A.C., and Myers, A.R. Aspirin-induced abnormalities of liver function. *Am J Dis Child.* 126:638–41, 1973.

22. Athreya, B.H., Moser, G., Cecil, H.S., and Myers, A.R. Aspirin-induced hepatotoxicity in JRA. A prospective study. *Arthritis Rheum.* 18:347–52, 1975.

23. Miller, J.J., III, and Weissman, D.B. Correlations between transaminase concentrations and serum salicylate concentrations in JRA. *Arthritis Rheum.* 19:115–18, 1976.

24. Seaman, W.E., and Platz, P.H. Effect of aspirin on liver tests in patients with RA or SLE and in normal volunteers. *Arthritis Rheum.* 19:155–60, 1976.

25. Koff, R.S., and Galdabini, J.J. Fever, myalgias, and hepatic failure in a 17 year old girl. *N Engl J Med.* 296:1337–47, 1977.

26. Sbarbaro, J.A., and Bennett, R.M. Aspirin hepatotoxicity and disseminated intravascular coagulation. *Ann Int Med.* 86:183–5, 1977.

27. Bywaters, E.G. The pathology of Still's Disease. Edited by M.I.V. Jayson. In *Still's Disease: Juvenile Chronic Polyarthritis.* New York: Academic Press, 1976.

28. Fassbender, H.G. *Pathology of Rheumatic Diseases.* New York: Springer-Verlag, 1975, pp. 186–8.

29. Schaller, J.G. Rheumatic diseases (inflammatory diseases of connective tissue, collagen diseases). Edited by V.C. Vaughn and R.J. McKay. In *Nelson: Textbook of Pediatrics.* Philadelphia: W.B. Saunders Co., 1975.

30. Scharf, J., Levy, J., Benderly, A., and Nakir, M. Pericardial tamponade in JRA. *Arthritis Rheum.* 19:760–2, 1976.

31. Sury, B., and Vesterdal, E. Extra-articular lesions in juvenile rheumatoid arthritis: a survey based upon a study of 151 cases. *Acta Rheum Scand.* 14:309–16, 1968.

32. Bywaters, E.G.L. Deaths in juvenile chronic polyarthritis. *Arthritis Rheum.* 20 (suppl):253–6, 1977.

33. Chylack, L., Bienfang, D., Bellows, R., and Stillman, J.S. Ocular manifestations of juvenile rheumatoid arthritis. *Am J Ophthalmol.* 79:1026–33, 1975.

34. Schaller, J.G. Iridocyclitis—informal discussion. *Arthritis Rheum.* 20 (suppl):227–30, 1977.

35. Jan, J.E., Hill, R.H., and Low, M.D. Cerebral complications in juvenile rheumatoid arthritis. *Can Med Assoc J.* 107:623–5, 1972.

36. Brown, G.L., and Wilson, W.P. Salicylate intoxication and the CNS with special reference to EEG findings. *Dis Nerv Syst.* 32:135–40, 1971.

37. Lang, H., Anttila, R., Svekus, A., and Laaksonen, A.-L. EEG findings in JRA and other connective tissue diseases in childhood. *Acta Ped Scand.* 63:373–80, 1974.

38. Petty, R.E., Cassidy, J., Burt, A., and Sullivan, D.B. Immunologic correlates of antinuclear antibody in juvenile rheumatoid arthritis, abstracted. *Arthritis Rheum.* 12:323, 1969.

39. Weinstein, M.P., and Hall, C.B. Mycoplasma pneumonia infection associated with migratory polyarthritis. *Am J Dis Child.* 127:125–6, 1974.

40. Fink, C., Windmiller, J., and Sartain, P. Arthritis as the presenting feature of childhood leukemia. *Arthritis Rheum.* 15:347–9, 1972.

41. Schaller, J.G. Arthritis as a presenting manifestation of malignancy in children. *J Pediatr.* 81:793–7, 1972.

42. Petty, R.E., Cassidy, J.T., and Sullivan, D.B. Serologic studies in juvenile rheumatoid arthritis: a review. *Arthritis Rheum.* 20 (suppl):260–7, 1977.

43. Calabro, J.J., Staley, H.L., Burnstein, S.L., and Leb, L. Laboratory findings in juvenile rheumatoid arthritis. *Arthritis Rheum.* 20 (suppl):268–9, 1977.

44. Calabro, J.J., Katz, A.M., and Maltz, B.A. A critical reappraisal of juvenile rheumatoid arthritis. *Clin Orthop.* 74:101–19, 1971.

45. Hanson, V., and Kornreich, H. Systemic rheumatic disorders ("collagen disease") in childhood: lupus erythematosus, anaphylactoid purpura, dermatomyositis, and scleroderma. *Bull Rheum Dis.* 17:435–46, 1967.

46. Cassidy, J.T., and Martel, W. Juvenile rheumatoid arthritis: Clinicoradiologic correlations. *Arthritis Rheum.* 20 (suppl):207–11, 1977.

47. Bernstein, B., Stobie, D., Singsen, B.H. et al. Growth retardation in juvenile rheumatoid arthritis (JRA). *Arthritis Rheum.* 20 (suppl):212–16, 1977.

10 Polyarticular Juvenile Rheumatoid Arthritis

Deborah W. Kredich

Polyarticular juvenile rheumatoid arthritis (JRA) is both the most common form of the disease and the one most likely to be diagnosed correctly. The definition of the polyarticular subtype of JRA has been varied and confusing in recent literature but current criteria define it as that with five or more involved joints during the initial six months of disease, excluding those patients with persistent, intermittent fevers to 39.5°C or those with rash.[1] Because of differences in reporting, it is difficult to determine the relative incidence of this group of patients. In most series 40% to 50% of all patients with JRA have a polyarticular onset, females outnumber males by nearly 2:1, and average age of onset is generally older than in the pauciarticular and systemic groups but with bimodal distribution peaking at ages one to three and eight to ten years.[2-7]

CLINICAL PRESENTATION

In this type of JRA joint disease usually overshadows the more general symptoms of illness. The usual presenting complaint is one of joint swelling and discomfort although the parents may have been aware of pallor, listlessness, anorexia, fever, or even weight loss prior to the point at which they appreciated joint symptoms. Stiffness on arising in the morning or after periods of inactivity during the day is a common complaint of older children with polyarticular-onset JRA. Younger children experience the same phenomenon but rarely complain so specific questioning by the physician relative to the types and speed of activities performed early in the morning may be needed. The duration of morning stiffness is often used as a parameter to gauge the activity of disease. Some children, especially younger ones, have little or no pain with their arthritis. Indeed, Scott and Ansell have recently reported studies of measurements of pain in children with arthritis and have found that severity of pain is significantly lower in children than in adults with rheumatoid arthritis.[8] In addition they found that severity of pain correlated poorly with other measures of disease activity and suggested that pain not be used as a parameter to assess treatment.

Although the larger joints, i.e., knees, wrists, and ankles, Figure 1, are commonly involved, symmetrical inflammation of the smaller, more distal joints is characteristic, Figure 2. One-fifth of the children have disease in the metacarpophalangeal (MCP) joints and in the proximal interphalangeal (PIP) joints. The metatarsals are also frequently affected. The cervical spine is often involved early and hip involvement is frequent at later stages. Less commonly, the temporomandibular, shoulder, sternoclavicular, cricoarytenoid, and distal interphalangeal (DIP) joints are affected. Cervical spine and large joint involvement are more common in children than in adults, but otherwise the pattern of joint disease is similar to that seen in adult rheumatoid arthritis.

The majority of children have swelling and tenderness of affected joints with effusions particularly common in the knees and wrists. Thickened synovial membranes may be appreciated as boggy swellings over the wrists, MCPs, PIPs, and sternoclavicular joints and as fullness at the elbows and around the ankles. Reflection of the synovial lining of the knee joint may be palpated by compressing it against underlying bony prominences of the femur on either side of the patella. Normal synovial reflection in childhood is about the thickness of a pencil lead while involved synovium may exceed the size of an average size pen in its reflection. Small effusions in the knee are best appreciated by eliciting a fluid wave and although larger effusions obscure this sign they do render the patella ballotable. Synovitis, with or without effusion, is often accompanied by increased warmth over the affected joint but erythema is much less common. Tenderness of the synovium may be elicited by lateral compression of PIP joints and of flexed MCP joints and may be the only sign of disease activity in these joints.

Although cervical spine disease may cause tenderness over the spine itself more commonly it produces pain on motion of the neck and results first in restriction of extension and lateral rotation. A significant amount of muscle spasm is often attendant.

Acute synovitis of the hip is difficult to assess clinically and involvement of the joint is inferred when motion produces pain. The hip

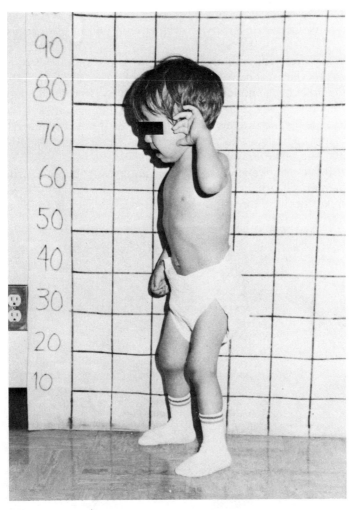

Figure 1. Photograph of 3-year-old boy with polyarticular JRA. He has swelling and contractures of both knees, contractures of his hips, and limited extension and rotation of his neck.

is held most comfortably in flexion and slight external rotation when inflammation is present. Hip pain is often referred to the groin or down to the knee (as may be pain from lower lumbar and sacral vertebrae, sacroiliac joints, and a number of pelvic structures). A sharp tap on the heel may produce immediate pain in the presence of synovitis, thus helping to localize the inflammation in confusing cases. X-rays are mandatory if an effusion is suspected, for the blood supply to the head of the femur is at risk if it remains untreated. Occasionally an arthrogram may be necessary.

Joint disease with synovial proliferation and effusions has been termed wet arthritis by some. A few children exhibit so-called dry arthritis. In these children onset of disease is commonly insidious and painless and the presence of flexion contractures in fingers or elbows is often the first change noticed by teachers and parents. Tenosynovitis is most frequent at wrists and ankles, usually, but not always, accompanying inflammation in the joints. Extensor and flexor tendon sheaths of the hand, peroneal and posterior tibial sheaths, and the Achilles' tendon at the ankle may be involved.

Systemic manifestations of disease are present but less striking in polyarticular JRA than in the systemic-onset form. Daily low-grade fever spikes occur in three-fourths of children at onset and accompany-

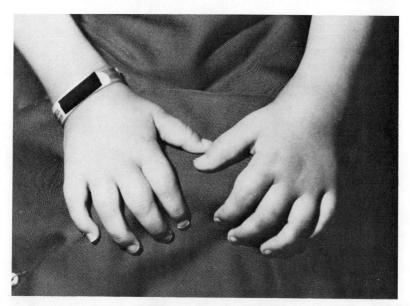

Figure 2. Photograph of hands of child shown in Figure 1. The wrists, metacarpophalangeal joints, and proximal interphalangeal joints are symmetrically swollen.

ing this are generalized malaise, anorexia, and sometimes weight loss.[9,10] Lymphadenopathy, while not as marked as in the systemic group, occurs in 40% of these patients, fewer have splenomegaly, and very few, hepatomegaly. Although most patients who develop iridocyclitis have a pauciarticular onset, approximately 14% of patients with a polyarticular onset have this manifestation sometimes occurring many years after disease onset.[11]

In contrast to the definition of disease onset-type in the current criteria,[1] Calabro[9] describes the rash of JRA in 19 of 48 patients with polyarticular onset. However, the rash is much more frequent in systemic-onset disease as are pleuritis, pericarditis and pneumonitis. The latter three entities are often asymptomatic and the true incidence is unknown, pleuritis being an incidental finding on chest x-ray. Bernstein found echocardiographic changes consistent with pericarditis in 36% of a group of JRA patients, over half of whom were not only asymptomatic but also had normal chest x-rays and ECGs.[12] In my experience diminished diffusion capacity has been noted in some patients.

Subcutaneous nodules occur more frequently with polyarticular disease than other forms.[9] As in adults with RA, nodules tend to occur in areas of pressure such as elbows, along the ulna, on the heels, and, in bedridden patients, on the occiput and along vertebrae. Nodules also occur in flexor tendons of the hands and feet. Pathologically they show less palisading and necrosis than those of adult rheumatoid arthritis, resembling more closely those of acute rheumatic fever.[13] Nodules are associated with positive latex fixation (LF) tests, erosive arthritis, and relatively poor prognosis, though none of these associations is absolute.[14]

Growth disturbances in JRA were described by Still in 1896.[15] Growth retardation occurs in two ways: generalized decrease in rate of growth as might be seen in any chronic disease; and localized growth disturbance secondary to specific joint involvement. Bernstein et al. have recently shown that overall growth is retarded less in polyarticular JRA than in the systemic type.[16] Localized undergrowth or overgrowth at epiphyses adjacent to involved joints is more obvious in pauciarticular disease, however, foreshortening of hands and feet secondary to involvement of carpals and tarsals occurs frequently in polyarticular disease. Additionally, Bernstein et al. found that a greater proportion of children with JRA than of normal children fall below the third percentile for height at onset of disease which may partially reflect the insidious nature of the onset, and partially parents' and physicians' inability to pinpoint date of onset.[16]

LABORATORY PARAMETERS

Many of the laboratory abnormalities in polyarticular JRA are less severe than those seen in systemic-onset disease. Anemia is relatively mild and may be of either the type associated with chronic disease and failure to utilize stored iron, or the anemia of iron deficiency secondary to salicylate-related gastrointestinal blood loss; a combination of the two is obviously possible. Older children with polyarticular disease rarely have hemoglobins less than 10g/dl; those under three yrs of age often do. Leukocytosis is also common, though white blood counts of greater than 20,000/mm³ are unusual. Thrombocytosis is occasionally seen and is thought to portend poor prognosis. Immunoglobulins are often increased in patients with polyarticular JRA.

Rheumatoid factor and fluorescent antinuclear antibody tests (FANA, ANA) are more frequently positive in polyarticular JRA than in the other onset-types.[17,18] Many investigators feel that the results of these tests have important associations with the natural history of the disease and the prognosis.[14,19] Hanson et al.[20] have shown that the positivity of the LF test for rheumatoid factor increases with age of onset of disease; that is, only 4% of children with onset of JRA under age four years are LF-positive, whereas 75% of children with onset ages of 12 to 16 years are LF-positive. In Hanson's group of polyarticular-onset patients, 52% were LF-positive while in most series only 10% to 15% of all JRA patients are LF-positive. Both Ansell[14] and Schaller[19] classify these seropositive patients separately and note that they have an older age of onset of disease, a higher percentage of nodules, a decreased frequency of control on aspirin therapy, and early evidence of erosive and severe progressive disease, particularly of the hands and feet.

Patients with earlier age of onset tend to have a higher incidence of ANA positivity.[17] The exact percentage of positives depends on the technique utilized, though many series agree that polyarticular-onset patients have a higher incidence of ANA positivity.[17,18] It is of interest that Schnitzer[21] has found ANA in very few of the patients developing amyloidosis and as with pauciarticular JRA, their presence is associated with development of uveitis.[11,22]

Cassidy and Sullivan have found that 4% of their JRA patients are IgA-deficient, deficiency being less common in the polyarticular-onset patients than in the pauciarticular-onset group.[23] It is important to recognize this subset of patients because they are susceptible to asthma and sinobronchial infections.

Liver enzyme abnormalities occur in JRA patients of all types. While aspirin hepatotoxicity has been implicated as the cause of elevated levels of serum transaminase by some, Rachelefsky et al.[24] and Miller et al.[25] have shown that elevations in SGOT may occur without relation to age, sex, or aspirin level, and that these levels may fall without change in aspirin dosage.

Urinary sediment abnormalities occur in JRA but significant renal involvement is not a feature of the disease. Up to one-fourth of all JRA patients in a recent study demonstrated hematuria or pyuria (defined as more than five cells per high-power field) in the absence of infection at some point in their disease.[26] Proteinuria occurred less frequently. A positive correlation between disease activity and pyuria or hematuria was noted, but increased numbers of white cells and red cells in the urine were also associated with aspirin therapy. A number of these children were biopsied, and 21% had mild abnormalities of numerous sorts, the most common being "local glomerulitis." The significance of this particular lesion is questionable since it was also noted in kidneys of "normal" children dying of trauma and other non-renal conditions. Renal function was rarely impaired except in patients developing amyloidosis. However, evaluation of the kidney during gold therapy becomes more difficult in view of these findings since the appearance of proteinuria or hematuria is usually thought to be an early sign of gold toxicity. Analgesic nephropathy may also occur, though the incidence is unknown.

The pathologic changes in the synovium of JRA are similar to those described in adult rheumatoid arthritis and are characterized by lymphocytic foci and plasma cell infiltration. However, the thick hyaline cartilage in children tends to protect the bone from erosion and may prolong the period during which recovery may occur. Because of this protective barrier, erosions tend to be marginal. Regenerative potential appears to exist in children since damaged hyaline cartilage is occasionally replaced by fibrocartilage thus restoring lost joint space.[27]

Radiologic changes in polyarticular JRA have been classified by Cassidy and Martel as early or advanced.[28] Soft tissue swelling and juxtaarticular osteoporosis are the main early changes. Periosteal new bone formation adjacent to involved joints is also seen in acute phases. Later changes in the polyarticular group include destruction of bone and cartilage, and eventually bony ankylosis. Cervical spine involvement occurs in 35% of polyarticular patients, and is manifest by fusion of the zygapophyseal joints, usually starting at C2-C3. Early appearance of erosions or bony defects in radiographs in children with arthritis should suggest nonrheumatologic conditions such as tumor or infection.

DIFFERENTIAL DIAGNOSIS

A complete list of conditions to be included in a differential diagnosis of polyarticular JRA might almost serve as a table of contents for a textbook on pediatrics. Features of a few of these conditions require amplification.

Acute rheumatic fever (ARF) presents the most common diagnostic dilemma with early polyarticular JRA. An unremitting fever pattern, exquisite joint tenderness, and prompt response to aspirin are features which favor a diagnosis of ARF over JRA in a patient with acute polyarticular arthritis. There are exceptions to each of these "rules," however, and diagnosis is only established with certainty after following some patients for weeks. The incidence of ARF has decreased markedly but varies with geography and socioeconomic environment and remains high in some areas. The clinical features of ARF have also changed with a decreasing incidence of carditis, chorea, nodules, and erythema marginatum;[29] consequently many cases have arthritis as the only major manifestation. Calabro has found that 30% of polyarticular JRA patients have persistently elevated antistreptolysin titers thus compounding the dilemma.[10] The patient's age is occasionally helpful since ARF is unusual under age four. Pericarditis without evidence of myocarditis or endocarditis favors a diagnosis of JRA as does involvement of the cervical spine. The rash may be confusing, but the macules in JRA are smaller and may occur on palms and soles. The rash of JRA, while evanescent over the course of the day, often recurs for weeks or months, while erythema marginatum rarely lasts over two weeks. The duration of joint manifestations, in the final analysis, makes clear the distinction between these two conditions, for joint symptoms in acute rheumatic fever usually last only a week or two and almost never over six weeks.[30]

Any of the rheumatic diseases can be associated with polyarthritis but systemic lupus erythematosus (SLE) and mixed connective tissue disease (MCTD) deserve particular mention. Arthritis and arthralgia are the most frequent presenting clinical manifestations of both and, though multisystem involvement is a hallmark of each, the clinical evolution may take months or years to become obvious. It is important to maintain vigilance and an openminded approach toward even the apparently straightforward polyarticular JRA patient. The onset of Raynaud's phenomenon in an arthritis patient should alert one to the possibility of MCTD, a syndrome characterized by a high titer of speckled ANA and antibodies to ribonucleoprotein (RNP).[31] In addition myositis, myocardial and pericardial disease, esophageal motility disturbances, renal disease, and sclerodermatous skin changes are clinical features suggestive of MCTD which might be overlooked if the index of suspicion is not high. Oral ulcers, alopecia, a positive Coombs' test, a false-positive serologic test for syphilis (STS), or urinary sediment abnormalities may be the first sign pointing to a diagnosis of SLE in a patient with polyarthritis. In both SLE and MCTD the importance of arriving at a diagnosis lies in appreciating the increased morbidity of the two diseases and realizing that more intensive treatment will be required.

Chronic inflammatory disease (ulcerative colitis and regional enteritis)[32] and psoriasis[33] are also associated with arthritis which may be polyarticular in presentation. Occasionally gastrointestinal symptoms in the inflammatory bowel diseases are subtle enough to be overshadowed by arthritis, especially if there is constipation rather than diarrhea. In these instances, marked growth retardation, anemia, mucosal ulcers or erythema nodosum in the presence of polyarthritis may be clues to the possibility of these diseases. In psoriasis, skin lesions may appear years after the arthritis or may be mild enough to remain undiagnosed. Nail pitting and involvement of DIP joints in a patient with polyarthritis are features favoring this diagnosis, and a positive family history for psoriasis may be helpful. Serum sickness reactions occurring in response to drugs, sera, or other toxins, are easily confused with early JRA. An urticarial skin eruption usually precedes joint effusions by several days. Joint pain and swelling are often marked, and fever is usual. Serum complement levels are usually decreased in serum sickness but normal or elevated in JRA.

Polyarticular arthritis or arthralgia may follow a large number of viral infections, best known of which is the arthritis of rubella infection, or that following rubella vaccination especially in teenage girls and young women.

MANAGEMENT

Specific aspects of drug treatment, physical therapy, and orthopedic intervention are covered in subsequent chapters. As the course of polyarticular disease is likely to be measured in terms of years, and possibilities for problems and complications are many it is in the best interest of the patient that one physician or group be responsible for overall management, although many specialists may be needed for optimal medical care. Some speciality examinations are required for all JRA patients on a relatively routine basis, and others are necessitated by the course of the disease. The most important example of the former is the ophthalmology examination and follow-up: the polyarticular-onset patient should be screened for iritis at time of diagnosis and every six months thereafter, until adulthood; orthopedists should be involved in longterm plans for reconstructive surgery; psychiatrists may be of help with some patients and families.

COMPLICATIONS

The possible complications attendant to polyarticular JRA are myriad. Most important are joint deformities secondary to bony destruction, soft tissue contractures, and growth disturbances. Loss of mobility of joints usually precedes evidence of bony fusion on radiographs and is caused by gradual shortening of muscles and tendons adjacent to inflamed joints which are allowed to assume a position of maximum comfort, usually flexion. Feet are held in plantar flexion and inversion. If physical therapy, splinting, and antiinflammatory measures are not adequate, fibrous or bony ankylosis occurs. The earliest losses are dorsiflexion of wrist and extension of neck. Subluxation of the ulna on the carpal bones and of C1 and C2 may occur, the latter possibly resulting in spinal cord damage in the event of trauma to the head or neck. After years of disease hips tend to dislocate or to develop *protrusio acetabuli*.[34] Osteoarthritis may occur in such hips in late teenage years or early adulthood. Prolonged contractures at large joints, particularly knees, and during periods of growth of adjacent long bones, allow for relative shortening of nerves and vessels in the area, thus complicating joint replacement surgery at the appropriate time. Inflammation in and around joints leads to shortening and contractures of some muscles and tendons, but laxity in other supporting juxtaarticular structures allowing for abnormal movements and for subluxations. This occurs commonly in the feet where the metatarsal heads sublux under the proximal portions of the phalanges producing a cocked-toe deformity. The resultant "rheumatoid foot" is difficult to fit comfortably into shoes, is subject to blisters, bunions, and painful calluses, and is a major cause of disability.[10]

Localized growth abnormalities produce numerous complications. Micrognathia occurs in at least 20% of patients and correlates closely with cervical spine involvement.[35] This condition results in severe orthodontic problems. Localized growth disturbances, asymmetric involvement of zygapophyseal joints, and muscle imbalance may play a part in development of scoliosis in 15% to 20% of patients.[35,36] Leg length inequality, a clue to asymmetry in the severity of involvement of joints, may lead to pelvic tilt, limp, and compensatory scoliosis. Vertebral collapse even in the absence of steroid therapy, occurs occasionally and must be considered in instances of posterior or radiating thoracic pain.

Sjogren's syndrome (keratoconjunctivitis sicca and xerostomia) occurs in a few patients with JRA, predominantly females with erosive arthritis, nodules, and positive LF tests.[37] Most have also had positive tests for ANA, normal serum complement, and no antibodies to DNA.[38] Onset of Sjogren's syndrome has been reported from two to 20 years after onset of arthritis. Visual loss and even blindness may result from iridocyclitis.

Vasculitis is a rarer complication of JRA than of adult rheumatoid arthritis. Secondary amyloidosis has been reported in as many as 7% of European JRA patients followed for 15 years[21] but the incidence in America and Australia appears far lower.[39] The earliest sign of amyloidosis is usually intermittent proteinuria, though diarrhea and abdominal pain, edema, and hypertension are common features at time of diagnosis. Of 51 patients with amyloidosis studied by Schnitzer and Ansell, 19 died, most with acute or chronic renal failure.[21] There is some evidence that treatment with chlorambucil ameliorates the proteinuria.

The psychosocial implications of JRA on the child as well as the family unit are enormous. As is true in any chronic disease for which there is no cure and no accurate prediction of outcome, parents have a mixture of guilt, anger, and anxiety. The children often learn to use their illness to manipulate the environment, selfimages are poor, and there are limitations, not only because of restrictions but also because of general fatiguability. Siblings often resent the time parents spend in the general care, physical therapy, and medical appointments for the child with arthritis.

The death rate in children with JRA is approximately 1% in the United States[39,40] and perhaps 4% in Europe,[41] the difference being due to infrequent occurrence of amyloidosis in American patients. Renal disease is the most frequent cause of death in European series and occurs primarily in patients who develop amyloidosis. The second most frequent cause of death in Europe and most common in the U.S. is infection. Hepatic failure is a prominent cause of death in several series.[40,42] Nearly all deaths occur in the polyarticular and systemic onset groups.

NATURAL HISTORY/PROGNOSIS

Accurate prediction regarding the duration of polyarticular disease and the ultimate degree of joint function is not possible at this time, a situation satisfying neither to parents nor physicians. The best that can be done is to rely on the data based on series concerning hundreds of patients at various intervals after onset. Some cases of polyarticular JRA have a monocyclic course with a good functional outcome, whereas others have a course marked by remissions and exacerbations, often with severe joint disability. Some have an unremitting course and a poor functional outcome.[10] Patients with seropositive polyarthritis tend to have a worse prognosis while a relatively large percentage of patients with seronegative polyarthritis have a good functional outlook.[19]

Two major parameters assessed at various intervals which provide some help in defining prognosis are the activity of joint inflammation and the functional capability of the patient. Criteria for activity of joint disease are the presence of effusion, soft tissue swelling, or pain on motion with limitation of motion. Disease activity overall tends to diminish over a period of years. However, roughly 30% of patients with polyarticular-onset disease will have disease activity 15 years after onset, not all with marked disability.[43] Overall prognosis in the majority of patients is good.[43,44]

It is hoped that continued research into etiology, natural history, and basic mechanisms of disease will make more accurate prediction of outcome for the individual patient a possibility in the future.

REFERENCES

1. Brewer, E.J., Jr., Bass, J., Baum, J. et al. Current proposed revision of JRA criteria. *Arthritis Rheum.* 20 (suppl):195–9, 1977.

2. Calabro, J.J., and Marchesano, J.M. The early natural history of juvenile rheumatoid arthritis. *Med Clin North Am.* 52:567–91, 1968.

3. Schaller, J., and Wedgwood, R.J. Juvenile rheumatoid arthritis: a review. *Pediatrics.* 50:940–53, 1972.

4. Goel, K.M., and Shanks, R.A. Follow-up study of 100 cases of JRA. *Ann Rheum Dis.* 33:25–31, 1974.

5. Bianco, A.J., and Peterson, H.A. JRA. *Orthop Clin North Am.* 2:745–59, 1971.

6. Sills, E.M. JRA and SLE in the adolescent. *Med Clin North Am.* 59:1497–1505, 1975.

7. Sullivan, D.B., Cassidy, J.T., and Petty, R.E. Pathogenic implications of age of onset in juvenile rheumatoid arthritis. *Arthritis Rheum.* 18:251–5, 1975.

8. Scott, P.J., Ansell, B.M., and Huskisson, E.C. Measurement of pain in juvenile chronic polyarthritis. *Ann Rheum Dis.* 36:186–7, 1977.

9. Calabro, J.J. Other extraarticular manifestations of juvenile rheumatoid arthritis. *Arthritis Rheum.* 20 (suppl):237–40, 1977.

10. Calabro, J.J., Holgerson, W.B., Sonpal, G.M., and Khoury, M.I. Juvenile rheumatoid arthritis: a general review and report of 100 patients observed for 15 years. *Semin Arthritis Rheum.* 5:257–98, 1977.

11. Chylack, L.T., Jr. The ocular manifestations of juvenile rheumatoid arthritis. *Arthritis Rheum.* 20 (suppl):217–23, 1977.

12. Bernstein, B., Takahashi, M., and Hanson, V. Cardiac involvement in JRA. *J Pediatr.* 85:313–17, 1974.

13. Bywaters, E.G.L., Glynn, L.E., and Zellis, A. Subcutaneous nodules of Still's disease. *Ann Rheum Dis.* 17:278–85, 1958.

14. Ansell, B.M., and Wood, P. Prognosis in juvenile chronic polyarthritis. *Clin Rheum Dis.* 2:397–412, 1976.

15. Still, G.F. A form of chronic joint disease in children. *Br Med J.* 2:1446–7, 1896.

16. Bernstein, B.H., Stoble, D., Singsen, B.H. et al. Growth retardation in juvenile rheumatoid arthritis. *Arthritis Rheum.* 20 (suppl):212–16, 1977.

17. Petty, R.E., Cassidy, J.T., and Sullivan, D.B. Clinical correlates of antinuclear antibodies in juvenile rheumatoid arthritis. *J Pediatr.* 83:386–98, 1973.

18. Hanson, V., Kornreich, H.K., Bernstein, B. et al. Three subtypes of juvenile rheumatoid arthritis. *Arthritis Rheum.* 20 (suppl):184–6, 1977.

19. Schaller, J.G. JRA: Series 1. *Arthritis Rheum.* 20 (suppl):165–70, 1977.

20. Hanson, V., Drexler, E., and Kornreich, H. The relationship of rheumatoid factor to age of onset in juvenile rheumatoid arthritis. *Arthritis Rheum.* 12:82–6, 1969.

21. Schnitzer, T.J., and Ansell, B.M. Amyloidosis in juvenile chronic polyarthritis. *Arthritis Rheum.* 20 (suppl):245–52, 1977.

22. Schaller, J.G., Johnson, G.D., Holborow, E.J. et al. The association of antinuclear antibodies with the chronic iridocyclitis of juvenile rheumatoid arthritis (Still's disease). *Arthritis Rheum.* 17:409–16, 1974.

23. Cassidy, J.T., Petty, R.E., and Sullivan, D.B. Occurrence of selective IgA deficiency in children with juvenile rheumatoid arthritis. *Arthritis Rheum.* 20 (suppl):181–3, 1977.

24. Rachelefsky, G.S., Kar, N., Coulson, A. et al. Serum enzyme abnormalities in juvenile rheumatoid arthritis. *Pediatrics.* 58:730–36, 1976.

25. Miller, J.J., III, and Weissman, D.B. Correlations between transaminase concentrations and serum salicylate concentration in juvenile rheumatoid arthritis. *Arthritis Rheum.* 19:115–18, 1976.

26. Anttila, R. Renal involvement in juvenile rheumatoid arthritis. *Acta Paediatr Scand.* 227 (suppl):1–73, 1972.

27. Bywaters, E.G.L. Pathologic aspects of juvenile chronic polyarthritis. *Arthritis Rheum.* 20 (suppl):271–8, 1977.

28. Cassidy, J.T., and Martel, W. JRA: clinicoradiologic correlations. *Arthritis Rheum.* 20 (suppl):207–11, 1977.

29. Markowitz, M. The changing picture of rheumatic fever. *Arthritis Rheum.* 20 (suppl):369–74, 1977.

30. Brewer, E.J., Jr. *Juvenile rheumatoid arthritis.* Philadelphia: W.B. Saunders Co., 1970.

31. Singsen, B.H., Bernstein, B.H., Kornreich, H.K. et al. Mixed connective tissue disease (MCTD) in childhood. A clinical and serologic study. *Pediatrics.* 90:893–900, 1977.

32. Schaller, J. Arthritis of inflammatory bowel disease. *Clin Rheum Dis.* 2:353–67, 1976.

33. Lambert, J., Ansell, B.M., Stephenson, E., and Wright, V. Psoriatic arthritis. *Clin Rheum Dis.* 2:339–59, 1976.

134

34. Rombouts, J.J., and Rombouts-Lindemanns, C. Involvement of the hip in juvenile rheumatoid arthritis. *Acta Rheum Scand.* 17:248–67, 1971.

35. Ansell, B.M. Joint manifestation in children with juvenile chronic polyarthritis. *Arthritis Rheum.* 20 (suppl):204–6, 1977.

36. Rombouts, J.J., and Rombouts-Lindemanns, C. Scoliosis in JRA. *J Bone Joint Surg.* 56-B:478–83, 1974.

37. Stillman, J.S., and Barry, P.E. JRA: Series 2. *Arthritis Rheum.* 20 (suppl):171–5, 1977.

38. Jackson, J., Anderson, L., Schur, P., and Stillman, J.S. Sjogren's syndrome in juvenile rheumatoid arthritis, abstracted. *Arthritis Rheum.* 16:122, 1973.

39. Baum, J., and Grazyna, G. Death in juvenile rheumatoid arthritis. *Arthritis Rheum.* 20 (suppl):253–7, 1977.

40. Bernstein, B.H. Death in juvenile rheumatoid arthritis. *Arthritis Rheum.* 20 (suppl):256–7, 1977.

41. Bywaters, E.G.L. Death in juvenile chronic polyarthritis. *Arthritis Rheum.* 20 (suppl):256, 1977.

42. Boone, J.E. Hepatic disease and mortality in juvenile rheumatoid arthritis. *Arthritis Rheum.* 20 (suppl):257–8, 1977.

43. Hanson, V., Kornreich, H.K., Bernstein, B.H. et al. Prognosis in juvenile rheumatoid arthritis. *Arthritis Rheum.* 20 (suppl):279–84, 1977.

44. Calabro, J.J., Stein, B., Staley, H.L., and Marchesano, J.M. Prognosis in juvenile rheumatoid arthritis. *Arthritis Rheum.* 20 (suppl):285, 1977.

11 Pauciarticular Juvenile Rheumatoid Arthritis

Carol B. Lindsley

The term pauciarticular is a word of Latin derivation, *paucus*, meaning a few and, *articulus*, meaning joint. It was first used by Green in 1940 to describe a type of childhood arthritis involving from two to four joints, while monarticular disease was considered a separate category.[1,2] However, more recently it has been used to include both monarticular and involvement up to five joints.[3] The 1976 Juvenile Rheumatoid Arthritis (JRA) Criteria Subcommittee definition is the one that will be used throughout this chapter,[4] i.e., one to four joints. Oligoarthritis is used synonymously by some authors.[5-7]

CLINICAL PRESENTATION

Pauciarticular-onset JRA encompasses 40% to 50% of all patients with JRA.[7-11] Single joint involvement or monarticular disease represents by itself 20% to 30% of JRA patients and approximately 50% to 60% of the pauciarticular group.[5,6] A majority of the monarticular patients will develop a pauciarticular pattern, frequently within weeks to months of disease onset and generally within one year; however, there appears to be no good reason to separate these two groups of patients as the nature of their disease and their prognosis appear to be the same.[3,7,12,13]

Age of Onset

The age of onset of pauciarticular arthritis ranges from six months to 15 years of age with peak ages being from one to four years.[8,13] The age limit of 15 years is arbitrary as this pattern has been reported in adulthood.[14] Griffin and coworkers[12] and more recently, Hanson et al.[11] reported that 50% to 57% respectively of their pauciarticular subtype were under four years of age at onset. Schaller[8] found a mean age of onset of 4.9 years and Fink,[10] a mean age onset of 5.8 years. A slightly later mean age of onset of seven years was reported by Calabro.[13]

General Appearance

The children with pauciarticular-onset disease are generally well and have normal growth and development. Occasionally mild systemic symptoms such as low-grade fever or malaise may be present.[3] Subcutaneous nodules are helpful diagnostically when present but are seldom seen in this group of patients and some studies report no patients with nodules and pauciarticular disease.[3]

Joint Pattern

Articular involvement may be acute but usually is insidious with varying degrees of pain, swelling, and/or limitation of motion. Palpable effusions as well as synovial thickening may contribute to the overall joint swelling. Lower extremity involvement may be heralded by antalgic limp. Severe hip pain may be present in contrast to the mild pain more commonly seen with other joints.

Large weight-bearing joints are usually the primary foci of the inflammatory activity and may be involved in an asymmetric pattern.[1,3] The knee is the most commonly involved of all joints[3,5] and is followed in frequency of involvement by other lower extremity joints, particularly ankle and hip.[13] Less frequent sites of involvement are the elbow, wrist and infrequently, single small joints of the hand or foot.[3,13] The distribution of involved joints in several studies is shown in Table 1. Hip involvement in the pauciarticular-onset group may indicate a likelihood of subsequent progression to polyarticular disease.[10]

Table 1
Pattern of Joint Involvement in Pauciarticular and Monarticular Arthritis

	Total No of Patients	Number of Joints					
		Knee	Hip	Wrist	Ankle	Elbow	Other‡
Cassidy[5]*	40	30	2	2	4	1	1
Calabro[6]*	32	14	5	0	4	3	6
Schaller[3]†	46	40	1	4	26	12	12
Griffin[12]*	39	27	5	2	3	1	1
Griffin[12]†	39	48	7	5	26	6	10
Bywaters and Ansell[15]*	33	23	0	2	5	0	3

*Patient populations having monarticular arthritis
†2 to 5 joints involved
‡Other joints: heel, MTP, PIP, toe, TMJ, C-spine, subtalar
Superscripts indicate references.

138

Sex

Bywaters and Ansell[15] did not find a difference in sex frequency in
their monarticular subtype, which was in contrast to findings in the systemic and polyarticular subtypes. In more recent reports children with
pauciarticular-onset disease have shown a mild to moderate female
predominance.[8,10,11] In addition, a highly significant difference in sex
distribution of certain subgroups within the pauciarticular-onset subtype has been reported. Specifically, a skewed sex distribution was
seen in young girls with pauciarticular-onset disease and iridocyclitis,
and boys with pauciarticular arthritis and the histocompatibility antigen
HLA-B27.[16] These two subgroups will be discussed more fully.

Laboratory Data

Laboratory data are not particularly helpful in making the diagnosis of
pauciarticular-onset JRA. The white blood cell count is generally in
normal range or mildly elevated. A mild anemia may be present during
active disease. The erythrocyte sedimentation rate ranges from normal
when the disease is inactive to markedly elevated during acute symptomatic exacerbations but is generally between 20 mm and 40mm/hr
(Westergren). The rheumatoid factor is rarely positive.[3,11] There may
be a mild hypergammaglobulinemia involving both the IgG and IgM
classes.[17]

Antinuclear antibodies (ANA) have been found to be present in
15% to 46% of patients with JRA and are present in a higher incidence
in the pauciarticular-onset subtype than in the systemic-onset subtype.[7,11] They are also present in a proportion in the polyarticular-onset
subtype which does not appear to differ significantly from that in the
pauciarticular-onset subtype.[11] ANA are mainly of the IgG class and
other autoantibodies, i.e., anti-DNA or anti-RNA have not been
found.[17] One recent study of immune complexes in JRA showed no
significant incidence of circulating immune complexes in the pauciarticular subtype in contrast to the systemic and polyarticular subtypes
of JRA.[18] LE cells are rarely if ever seen in the pauciarticular-onset
patients.[3]

Histocompatibility antigens in JRA have been studied recently
and the HLA-B27 antigen has been demonstrated to have a particularly
high incidence in boys with pauciarticular disease, in one study representing 60% of this subgroup.[16]

Joint fluid findings do not differ significantly from those seen in
polyarticular disease. Generally, a class II (inflammatory) fluid is pres-

ent, manifested by a leukocytosis, increased protein and mildly decreased synovial fluid glucose.[5,6,19] There is a poor correlation between the degree of leukocytosis and the clinical presence of active disease.[5] Griffin reported 62% with a fair mucin clot and 23% with a poor one.[12] The total hemolytic complement (CH50) generally is normal to slightly decreased in the synovial fluid and the serum complement values are in the normal range.[20]

Synovial Histology

The histologic findings are less severe in pauciarticular disease than those seen in the other JRA subtypes. There is nonspecific synovitis with synovial cell hypertrophy and lymphocytic and occasionally plasma cell infiltrates.[5] There is also increased vascularity and tissue edema. The marginal pannus and lymphocytic foci seen in seropositive disease and in adult rheumatoid arthritis may be seen occasionally.[21]

X-ray Findings

Radiographic findings vary depending on the disease duration and severity. Early in disease there is only soft-tissue swelling and juxtaarticular demineralization which may be the only findings for months to years after disease onset. With progression of disease there may be loss of joint space and erosions but severe destructive changes or ankylosis are unusual. If severe destructive changes do occur they are usually in the hip or shoulder.[22] In a report dealing with monarticular JRA, 11 of 40 patients had evidence of bone erosions.[5] Abnormalities in bone growth may also be seen on radiographs and include accelerated epiphyseal maturation, metaphyseal overgrowth, and longitudinal overgrowth of the long bones.[5] Periostitis is also a frequent finding.[22]

DIFFERENTIAL DIAGNOSIS

To meet the most recent proposed criteria for diagnosis of pauciarticular-onset JRA, arthritis must persist for at least six weeks in one to four joints when other subtypes are excluded.[4] In addition a long list of other diseases must be excluded; this list varies according to overall duration of symptoms and the initial joint involved. Definite early diagnosis of monarticular involvement is particularly difficult and requires synovial fluid analysis or synovial biopsy.

Infectious Arthritis

A primary concern in the differential list is infectious arthritis particularly in monarticular disease of less than three months' duration, as a slowly smoldering bacterial, tuberculous, or fungal arthritis can present in such a manner. In general infected joints are severely painful with marked erythema and tenderness. The patient is usually febrile and has a history of acute onset of pain or loss of function. However, if the infection is produced by a mildly pathogenic organism, or the clinical course is modified by partial antibiotic therapy, clinical symptoms may be less severe. Synovial fluid analysis and culture in monarticular disease are critical. Occasionally synovial biopsy is also required to exclude tuberculous or fungal arthritis, which in the case of the former, has granulomas and giant cells.[23] The synovial fluid in infectious arthritis is usually cloudy or turbid with a poor mucin clot and there is a marked leukocytosis in the range of 50,000 to greater than 100,000 cells per cu mm.[19] A gram stain of the synovial fluid may reveal organisms. Blood cultures increase the chance of identification of the etiologic agent by another 20%, being positive in 60% to 80% of patients with septic arthritis.[24,25] Synovial fluid glucose is usually markedly reduced in septic arthritis, being more than 50 mg% below the blood glucose level.[19]

Viral arthritis may accompany several of the childhood diseases such as rubella, chickenpox, mumps. In addition, viral hepatitis in teenagers may cause arthritis.[26] However, viral arthritis is usually of less than two weeks' duration and accompanied by other signs of viral disease, e.g., characteristic exanthem.

Other Types of Rheumatic Arthritis

a) Ankylosing spondylitis: Approximately 20% of ankylosing spondylitis begins with peripheral arthritis.[27-29] Early in the disease before there is evidence of sacroiliac or lumbar spine involvement, it may be impossible to exclude this diagnosis. However, diagnosis is clarified if one finds clinical or radiographic evidence of lumbodorsal spine involvement and radiographic changes in the sacroiliac joints.[27,29]

b) Systemic lupus erythematosus: This disease frequently presents with inflammatory arthritis but can be excluded by a negative antinuclear antibody test and by the absence of other clinical and laboratory criteria.[30]

c) Rheumatic fever: The arthritis seen in rheumatic fever is usually of less than six weeks' duration and has a migratory pattern with severe pain accompanying the initial episode. This diagnosis also requires evidence of recent streptococcal disease—positive throat culture for beta-hemolytic streptococci, or four-fold increase in ASO titer, or other antistreptococcal antibody titers.[31]

d) Vasculitis: Vasculitic syndromes present a spectrum of disease including anaphylactoid purpura, polyarteritis, hypersensitivity, and allergic reactions. All of these have underlying systemic disease and frequently have cutaneous or mucocutaneous lesions which are diagnostic. Anaphylactoid purpura (Schoenlein-Henoch purpura) has a characteristic purpuric rash distributed over the extensor aspect of the lower extremities and frequently has associated abdominal pain. This is the most common of the vasculitides in the pediatric age group. In infants the recently described mucocutaneous lymph node syndrome which resembles infantile polyarteritis should also be considered.[32]

Less common rheumatic disorders such as scleroderma, psoriatic arthritis and Reiter's disease can be excluded on a clinical basis. Polymyositis/dermatomyositis not uncommonly is associated with arthritis but presents with systemic symptoms and symmetrical proximal muscle weakness.

Orthopedic Disorders

A variety of orthopedic disorders and mechanical problems can present as monarticular disease. These can usually be distinguished on clinical and radiographic findings and include osteochondritis, toxic synovitis (observation hip), Legg-Perthés disease, slipped capital femoral epiphysis, trauma, chondromalacia patellae syndrome, and numerous congenital anomalies.

Miscellaneous

This group includes inflammatory bowel disease, neoplastic and hematologic diseases, villonodular synovitis, and sarcoidosis which must be excluded by a combination of clinical findings and laboratory data.

SUBGROUPS

There are at least two subgroups within the pauciarticular-onset subtype that deserve special attention. Each has an immunologic marker, particular risks, and prognosis. These are 1) boys with pauciarticular arthritis and associated histocompatibility antigen HLA-B27 (formerly W-27), who are at risk for developing ankylosing spondylitis, and 2) girls with pauciarticular arthritis, antinuclear antibodies, and a high risk for developing chronic iridocyclitis.

The histocompatibility system of antigens is a major factor in graft rejection. Serologic typing of these antigens has become available in recent years. In 1973 Brewerton and colleagues found that the HLA-B27 antigen was present in over 90% of patients with ankylosing spondylitis.[33] Subsequently, associations have been sought between this antigen and other rheumatic diseases. In 1974 several reports appeared noting an overall increased incidence of HLA-B27 in juvenile rheumatoid arthritis.[34-36] In addition, long term studies had indicated that from 5% to 8% of children with JRA developed ankylosing spondylitis.[29,37] One study demonstrated over half the children had experienced peripheral arthritis preceding spinal involvement from two to 13 years before evidence of lumbar spine disease.[28] The ankylosing spondylitis occurred in boys with lower limb involvement and late-onset JRA and was indistinguishable in its early phases from pauciarticular-onset JRA.

The initial report of the incidence of HLA-B27 antigen in JRA dealt with a relatively small group of patients and reported a 42% incidence in contrast to 6% incidence in the control population.[36] This early study found no predilection for specific subtypes of JRA but did note increased frequency of seronegativity and involvement of males in their HLA-B27–positive patients. A series of conflicting reports has appeared.[34,35,39] The most recent and largest studies are from Boston, 123 patients,[40] and Seattle, 121 patients.[16] In the first study a 15% incidence of HLA-B27 antigen was identified in a patient population screened to remove those with sacroiliitis and this was not significantly increased over their controls of 6%. In the Seattle study a 26% incidence of HLA-B27 antigen was seen in the entire series. However, on careful scrutiny it was found that this higher incidence was accounted for by an increase in two subgroups: a) boys with pauciarticular disease (61%) and, b) children who had subsequently developed ankylosing spondylitis (100%). These two groups also included 12 of the 14 patients in the entire series with bilateral sacroiliitis. The patients were seronegative and had no antinuclear antibodies. (See Chapter 8.)

The second subgroup that has been noted is that of young girls with pauciarticular-onset disease and chronic iridocyclitis. The general incidence of iridocyclitis in JRA is reported from 8% to 34% and averages approximately 10%.[3,41-43] The fact that patients with the least arthritis had the greatest incidence of eye disease has been recently emphasized by Schaller, et al.[44,45] who called attention to a 29% incidence of iridocylitis in children with pauciarticular-onset subtype. Subsequently the range in the pauciarticular subtype has been reported to be from 16% to 34% in different series.[7-11] Seventy-five percent to 95% of all iridocyclitis occurred in patients with pauciarticular-onset disease.[42-46] In this subtype there is a female predominance which persists in the patients that have iridocyclitis.[16] Chronic iridocyclitis occurs infrequently in the polyarticular subtype and rarely in systemic disease.

Arthritis generally precedes eye disease from one to 10 years but can follow iridocyclitis by months to years.[41,44-46] The eye disease is insidious and asymptomatic in a majority but can be accompanied by one or more symptoms such as photophobia, excess tearing, redness, or pain. One or both eyes may be affected with reports of bilateral eye disease ranging from 33% to greater than 50%.[41,44,47] There appears to be no relationship between the activity of arthritis and that of eye disease.[42]

In Chylack's study 69% of the arthritis ultimately associated with iridocyclitis had its onset under four years of age. The age of onset of eye disease ranged from three to 16 years with 19% occurring under age four.[42] Smiley reported an average age of onset for arthritis of 3.9 years and for eye disease of seven years.[43] The exact onset of eye disease is difficult to ascertain given the frequent insidious nature of the lesion.

The association of iridocyclitis with antinuclear antibodies has been noted, the exact incidence varying according to the method used for detection of the antibodies.[17,48] A positive ANA can serve as a practical indicator of patients with increased risk for chronic iridocyclitis: Schaller and associates found an 88% incidence of positive ANAs in their patients with eye disease.[17]

This represents the prime cause of morbidity in the pauciarticular arthritis group. Of those with eye involvement, 50% or more may have permanent visual impairment,[43] the actual cause being glaucoma, band keratopathy, cataract, adhesions involving the uveal tract, or combination thereof.[42]

This chronic disease differs significantly from acute iridocyclitis, which is associated with ankylosing spondylitis and occurs primarily in males with later onset of arthritis. Acute iridocyclitis has definite symptoms associated with the inflammatory condition and there appears to be little or no long term morbidity from it. (See Chapter 12.)

NATURAL HISTORY

The pauciarticular disease pattern persists in at least 66% of those who manifest this mode of onset. In the remaining group progression to polyarticular involvement occurs. In Green's initial report on pauciarticular disease involving 35 children, 9% went on to develop a polyarticular pattern.[1] More recently Fink[10] reported progression to polyarticular involvement in 36% and Calabro[13] in 25% of those with a pauciarticular-onset pattern. In the group with only single joint involvement initially, a majority progressed to pauciarticular involvement and relatively few to polyarticular involvement. The exact distribution of these patients with monarticular onset and their subsequent course is outlined in Table 2. Laaksonen found persistent monarticular disease in only four of 485 patients.[49]

The clinical course is characterized by numerous exacerbations and remissions. Although many will have continued disease activity after five to 25 years, there is usually little functional impairment of the involved joints.[50-54] About one-half will experience long term remission.[13] The pauciarticular-onset subtype has a better functional outcome than either the polyarticular- or the systemic-onset subtypes.[7,52]

Disability is determined by the actual number of joints involved, disease duration and severity, appropriateness of therapy, and duration of disease at the time of referral to a multidisciplinary center.[9] In Griffin's study, nine of 27 patients with disease duration greater than two years had functional residua.[1] None of Calabro's[51] "oligoarthritis" group were in the ARA functional class III or IV,[55] and Schaller[3] reported no severe disability in 32 patients with pauciarticular disease; joint destruction was infrequent in both studies. In a 30-year follow-up study, 45% of the pauciarticular onset group were in functional class I and only 10% were disabled (ARA class III or IV).[1,7] Adequate

Table 2
Course of Monarticular Onset Arthritis

	Total Number of Patients	Persistent Monarticular Disease	Developed Pauciarticular Disease	Developed Polyarticular Disease
Griffin[12]	39	0	38	1
Calabro[6]	32	2	22	8
Cassidy[5]	40	9	19	12
Bywaters and Ansell[15]	33	14	7	14*

*Included four joints or more
Superscripts indicate references.

nonsteroidal antiinflammatory medication, local joint care and protection, and appropriate exercises are critical in preventing disability. (See Chapters 14 and 15.)

Complications from the joint disease itself are relatively mild. These include growth disturbances and occasionally joint destruction. Growth disturbances may be a leg-length anomaly with either epiphyseal overgrowth producing increased length on the involved side or premature epiphyseal closure resulting in a shortened limb.[22,53] These discrepancies may disappear when the disease is in remission although they occasionally result in permanent deformity and necessitate surgical intervention. Ligamentous laxity from chronic inflammation may further exaggerate functional problems originally caused by abnormal growth patterns. For example, severe genu valgus may be a combination of medial epiphyseal overgrowth and ligamentous laxity. Flexion contractures frequently seen in long-standing disease can usually be prevented if aggressive physical and medical therapy are instituted early in the disease course. (See Chapters 15 and 16.)

REFERENCES

1. Green, W.T. Monoarticular and pauciarticular arthritis in children. *JAMA*. 115:2023–36, 1940.

2. Schaller, J., and Wedgwood, R.J. Classification of juvenile rheumatoid arthritis. *N Engl J Med*. 277:1374, 1967.

3. Schaller, J., and Wedgwood, R.J. Juvenile rheumatoid arthritis: a review. *Pediatrics*. 50:940–53, 1972.

4. Brewer, E.J., Jr., Bass, J., Baum, J. et al. Current proposed revision of JRA criteria. *Arthritis Rheum*. 20 (suppl):195–9, 1977.

5. Cassidy, J.T., Brody, G.L., and Martel, W. Monarticular juvenile rheumatoid arthritis. *J Pediatr*. 70:867–75, 1967.

6. Calabro, J.J., Parino, G.R., and Marchesano, J.M. Monarticular-onset juvenile rheumatoid arthritis. *Bull Rheum Dis*. 21:613–16, 1970.

7. Stillman, J.S., and Barry, P.E. Juvenile rheumatoid arthritis: Series 2. *Arthritis Rheum*. 20 (suppl):171–5, 1977.

8. Schaller, J.G. Juvenile rheumatoid arthritis: Series 1. *Arthritis Rheum*. 20 (suppl):165–70, 1977.

9. Ansell, B.M. Juvenile chronic polyarthritis: Series 3. *Arthritis Rheum*. 20 (suppl):176–7, 1977.

10. Fink, C.W. Patients with JRA: a clinical study. *Arthritis Rheum*. 20 (suppl):183–4, 1977.

11. Hanson, V., Kornreich, H.K., Bernstein, B. et al. Three subtypes of juvenile rheumatoid arthritis: correlations of age at onset, sex, and serologic factors. *Arthritis Rheum*. 20 (suppl):184–6, 1977.

12. Griffin, P.P., Tachdjian, M.O., and Green, W.T. Pauciarticular arthritis in children. *JAMA*. 184:145–50, 1963.

13. Calabro, J.J., and Marchesano, J.M. The early natural history of juvenile rheumatoid arthritis. *Med Clin North Am*. 52:567–91, 1968.

146

14. Bywaters, E.G.L. Still's disease in the adult. *Ann Rheum Dis.* 30:121–33, 1971.

15. Bywaters, E.G.L., and Ansell, B.M. Monoarticular arthritis in children. *Ann Rheum Dis.* 24:116–22, 1965.

16. Schaller, J.G., Ochs, H.D., Thomas, E.D. et al. Histocompatibility antigens in childhood-onset arthritis. *J Pediatr.* 88:926–30, 1976.

17. Schaller, J.G., Johnson, G.D., Holborow, E.J. et al. The association of antinuclear antibodies with the chronic iridocyclitis of juvenile rheumatoid arthritis (Still's Disease). *Arthritis Rheum.* 17:409–16, 1974.

18. Person, D.A., Brewer, E.J., and Rossen, R.D. Immune complexes and antinuclear antibodies in sera from patients with juvenile rheumatoid arthritis, abstracted. *Clin Res.* 25:365A, 1977.

19. Jessar, R.A. The study of synovial fluids. Edited by J.L. Hollander, and D.J. McCarty, Jr. In *Arthritis and Allied Conditions.* 8th ed. Philadelphia: Lea & Febiger Publishers, 1972, pp. 67–81.

20. Bianco, N.E., Panush, R.S., Stillman, J.S., and Schur, P.H. Immunologic studies in juvenile rheumatoid arthritis. *Arthritis Rheum.* 14:685–96, 1971.

21. Bywaters, E.G.L. Pathologic aspects of juvenile chronic polyarthritis. *Arthritis Rheum.* 20 (suppl):271–6, 1977.

22. Ansell, B.M. Joint manifestations in children with juvenile chronic polyarthritis. *Arthritis Rheum.* 20 (suppl):204–6, 1977.

23. Amberson, J.B., Jr. Pathogenesis and medical treatment of tuberculosis of vertebrae. *J Bone Joint Surg.* 22:807–14, 1940.

24. Nelson, J.D., and Koontz, W.D. Septic arthritis in infants and children: a review of 117 cases. *Pediatrics.* 38:966–71, 1966.

25. Almquist, E.E. The changing epidemiology of septic arthritis in children. *Clin Orthop.* 68:96–9, 1970.

26. Phillips, P.E. Viral arthritis in children. *Arthritis Rheum.* 20 (suppl):584–9, 1977.

27. Schaller, J., Bitnum, S., and Wedgwood, R.J. Ankylosing spondylitis with childhood onset. *J Pediatr.* 74:505–16, 1969.

28. Ladd, J.R., Cassidy, J.T., and Martel, W. Juvenile ankylosing spondylitis. *Arthritis Rheum.* 14:579–90, 1971.

29. Jacobs, P. Ankylosing spondylitis in children and adolescents. *Arch Dis Child.* 38:492–9, 1963.

30. Systemic Lupus Erythematosus Criteria Subcommittee of the American Rheumatism Association Section of the Arthritis Foundation: Preliminary criteria for the classification of systemic lupus erythematous. *Bull Rheum Dis.* 21:643–8, 1973.

31. Council on Rheumatic Fever and Congenital Heart Disease of the American Heart Association: Jones criteria (revised) for guidance in the diagnosis of rheumatic fever. *Circulation.* 32:664, 1965.

32. Kawasaki, T., Kasaki, F., Okawa, S. et al. A new infantile acute febrile mucocutaneous lymph node syndrome prevailing in Japan. *Pediatrics.* 54:271–6, 1974.

33. Brewerton, D.A., Caffrey, M., Hart, F.D. et al. Ankylosing spondylitis and HL-A27. *Lancet.* 1:904–7, 1973.

34. Buc, M., Nyulassy, S., Stefanovic, J. et al. HL-A system and juvenile rheumatoid arthritis. *Tissue Antigens.* 4:395–7, 1974.

35. Edmonds, J., Morris, R.I., Metzger, A.L. et al. Follow-up study of juvenile chronic polyarthritis with particular reference to histocompatibility antigen W27. *Ann Rheum Dis.* 33:289–92, 1974.

36. Rachelefsky, G.S., Terasaki, P.I., Katz, R., and Stiehm, E.R. Increased prevalence of W27 in juvenile rheumatoid arthritis. *N Engl J Med.* 290:892–4, 1974.

37. Carter, M.E. Sacroiliitis in Still's Disease. *Ann Rheum Dis.* 21:105–20, 1962.

38. Ansell, B.M., and Bywaters, E.G.L. Diagnosis of "probable" Still's disease and its outcome. *Ann Rheum Dis.* 21:253–62, 1962.

39. Hall, M.A., Ansell, B.M., James, D.C.O., and Zylinski, P. HL-A antigens in juvenile chronic polyarthritis (Still's disease). *Ann Rheum Dis.* 34 (suppl):36–8, 1975.

40. Gibson, D.J., Carpenter, C.B., Stillman, J.S., and Schur, P.H. Reexamination of histocompatibility antigens found in patients with juvenile rheumatoid arthritis. *N Engl J Med.* 293:636–8, 1975.

41. Calabro, J.J., Parrino, R., Atchoo, P.D. et al. Chronic iridocyclitis in juvenile rheumatoid arthritis. *Arthritis Rheum.* 13:406–13, 1970.

42. Chylack, L.T., Bienfang, D.C., Bellows, A.R., and Stillman, J.S. Ocular manifestations of juvenile rheumatoid arthritis. *Am J Ophthalmol.* 79:1026–33, 1975.

43. Smiley, W.K. The eye in juvenile rheumatoid arthritis. *Trans Ophthalmol Soc UK.* 94:817–29, 1974.

44. Schaller, J., Kupfer, C., and Wedgwood, R.J. Iridocyclitis in juvenile rheumatoid arthritis. *Pediatrics.* 44:92–100, 1969.

45. Schaller, J., Smiley, W.K., and Ansell, B.M. Iridocyclitis of juvenile rheumatoid arthritis (JRA, Still's disease): a follow-up study of 76 patients, abstracted. *Arthritis Rheum.* 16:130, 1973.

46. Jose, D.G., and Good, R.A. Iridocyclitis and pauciarticular juvenile rheumatoid arthritis. *J Pediatr.* 78:910–11, 1971.

47. Smiley, W.K. The visual prognosis in Still's disease with eye involvement, abstracted. *Proc Roy Soc Med.* 53:196, 1960.

48. Petty, R.E., Cassidy, J.T., and Sullivan, D.B. Clinical correlates of antinuclear antibodies in juvenile rheumatoid arthritis. *J Pediatr.* 83:386–9, 1973.

49. Laaksonen, A.-L. A prognostic study of juvenile rheumatoid arthritis: analysis of 544 cases. *Acta Paediatr Scand.* 166:1–168, 1966.

50. Hanson, V., Kornreich, H., Bernstein, B. et al. Prognosis of juvenile rheumatoid arthritis. *Arthritis Rheum.* 20 (suppl):279–84, 1977.

51. Calabro, J.J., Burnstein, S.L., Staley, H.L., and Marchesano, J.M. Prognosis in juvenile rheumatoid arthritis: a fifteen-year follow-up of 100 patients. *Arthritis Rheum.* 20 (suppl):285, 1977.

52. Calabro, J.J., and Marchesano, J.M. Prognosis in juvenile rheumatoid arthritis, abstracted. *Arthritis Rheum.* 8:434, 1965.

53. Ansell, B.M., and Bywater, E.G.L. Prognosis in Still's disease. *Bull Rheum Dis.* 9:189–91, 1959.

54. Goel, K.M., and Shanks, R.A. Follow-up study of 100 cases of juvenile rheumatoid arthritis. *Ann Rheum Dis.* 33:25–31, 1974.

55. Steinbrocker, O., Traeger, C.H., and Batteiman, R.C. Therapeutic criteria in rheumatoid arthritis. *JAMA.* 140:569–662, 1949.

12 Ocular Manifestations of Juvenile Rheumatoid Arthritis: Pathology, Fluorescein Iris Angiography, and Patient Care Patterns

Leo T. Chylack, Jr.,
David K. Dueker, and
Donovan J. Pihlaja

In spite of recent successes in reducing the incidence of blinding complications of juvenile rheumatoid arthritis, we still are totally ignorant of many of the most basic characteristics of the ocular syndrome.[1-5]

We have assumed that ocular manifestations of JRA are inflammatory, hence the term uveitis. However, we have no pathologic or other evidence that inflammation is restricted to the iris (iritis) or the iris-ciliary body (iridocyclitis). Only three authors have reported abnormalities of the posterior segment; inflammatory cells in the retrolental vitreous,[6] choroidal inflammation,[7] retinal scar,[8] and papillitis/papilledema.[4,5] The scarcity of tissue for pathologic study and the reluctance of investigators to take aqueous humor samples from JRA patients with iridocyclitis has perpetuated our ignorance about this syndrome. Even several comprehensive clinical studies have not yielded a consistent picture of the ocular problems of JRA.[1-5] Patient populations are not consistently derived or defined. Some include ankylosing spondylitics[9] in spite of the exclusion of this disease from the criteria accepted by the American Rheumatism Association.[10]

149

Others contain disproportionately large numbers of advanced cases and not surprisingly, report poor therapeutic results and a pessimistic view of this disease.[3] Even those authors reporting good therapeutic results are uncertain about exactly which factor in their approach is responsible for their success.[1,2,4,5]

It is the purpose of this chapter 1) to present the pathology of the iris in JRA from specimens obtained at cataract surgery, 2) report the preliminary results of fluorescein iris angiography in JRA, a technique which offers us a new and broader understanding of the anterior segment inflammation, and 3) to review some of the basic patterns of health care being provided by rheumatologists and ophthalmologists working with JRA patients. Some of the recent advances in immunology and genetics will also be mentioned as well as some suggestions for future clinical and laboratory research efforts.

PATHOLOGY

All the iris specimens we have studied were obtained at the time of peripheral iridectomy during elective cataract extraction. One was fixed in 10% formalin, routinely embedded in paraffin, sectioned and stained with hemotoxylin and eosin. The other two specimens were fixed in 2.5% buffered glutaraldehyde and postfixed with 1% buffered osmium tetroxide; the buffering conditions used were 0.15M phosphate buffer at pH 7.3 (22°C). After fixation the specimens were dehydrated with 2,2-dimethoxypropane, embedded in Epon, sectioned at 1μm and stained with toluidine blue.[11] All specimens were observed and photographed with a Carl Zeiss Photomicroscope III (7082 Oberkochen, West Germany).

The patients' histories were as follows:

Case 1. P.J. was a 58-year-old white female with polyarticular JRA with no clinical history of iritis. Cataracts developed at age 49 and were posterior subcapsular in type. The iris was completely normal on slit-lamp examination. The specimen was from a basal sector iridectomy.

Case 2. K.B. was a 13-year-old white female with pauciarticular JRA who had severe bilateral iridocyclitis with onset in both eyes (OU) at approximately six years of age. Chronic steroid and mydriatic therapy was necessary for several years. A mature cataract developed in the left eye (OS) and then shrunk to a thickened lens remnant which was removed intact at age 13. The specimen was from a large peripheral iridectomy. No active inflammation was present at time of surgery.

Case 3. L.L. was a 9-year-old white female with polyarticular JRA who was found to have active iridocyclitis OU at age five years.

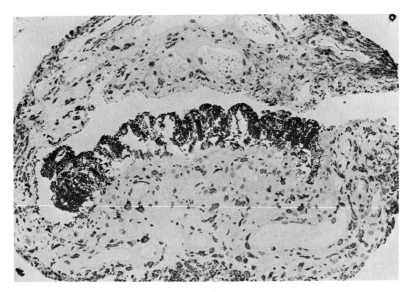

Figure 1. Photomicrograph of peripheral iridectomy specimen from patient L.L. Specimen appears normal except for increase in vascularity. Formalin-fixed, epon-embedded. Toluidine-blue, 270X. Marker = 50μM.

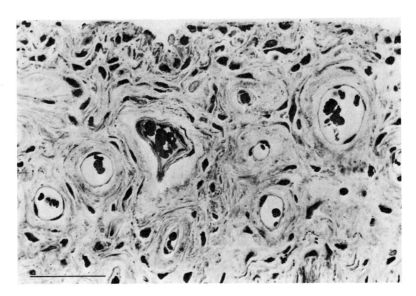

Figure 2. Photomicrograph of peripheral iridectomy specimen from patient K.B. Vessels are normal but there is round cell infiltrate along anterior surface of iris. Glutaraldehyde-fixed, epon-embedded. Toluidine-blue, 640X. Marker = 50μM.

Except for posterior synechiae OS, eyes were normal with visual acuity of 20/20 OU. She had recurrent intermittently active iridocyclitis OU requiring frequent topical steroids and mydriatics. A peculiar cortical snowflake cataract developed at age seven and progressed to significant visual loss (20/140-20/400) by age eight and one-half years. At time of phacoaspiration with a Cavitron phacoemulsifier the iridocyclitis was quiescent. The specimen of iris was peripheral.

All three specimens show surprisingly few abnormalities. The basic structural components of the iris appear to be intact, Figure 1. The iris vessels may be slightly increased in number, particularly in patient L.L., Figure 1, but this may be more characteristic of the young age of the patient than of any JRA-related change and was not seen in the other two specimens. The other features of the iris appear to be normal, Figure 2. The cells populating the iris appear to be normal in number and type, but in a few sections there was a round-cell infiltrate along the anterior surface of the iris. The pigmented epithelial layers of the iris appear to be normal, Figure 3. These specimens do not indicate the source of the inflammatory cells seen in the aqueous humor in this disease, nor do they by virtue of their origin allow us to examine the nature of the posterior synechial adhesions which occur in 26% of patients with iridocyclitis.[5] Possibly specimens obtained from the pupillary zone in acutely inflamed eyes would be more informative.

Thus pathologic changes noted in these three patients at the time of elective cataract surgery were not particularly revealing. Only one patient was free of ocular inflammation in the operated eye for several years; the remaining two, albeit quiescent at the time of surgery, had had prior months of persistent low-grade inflammation. The lack of significant inflammatory infiltrate was surprising. Further study is not only desirable but quite feasible now that cataract surgery is achieving greater success. A larger number of iridectomy specimens studied with electron microscopy or with immunological techniques might enhance our understanding of the iridocyclitis.

FLUORESCEIN ANGIOGRAPHY*

All patients with iridocyclitis and JRA in the population under study at the Robert Breck Brigham Hospital except those under the age of seven years or living great distances from Boston were considered for

*The assistance of Joan L. Nobel, M.D. with the protocol for and the performance of the fluorescein iris angiograms is gratefully acknowledged.

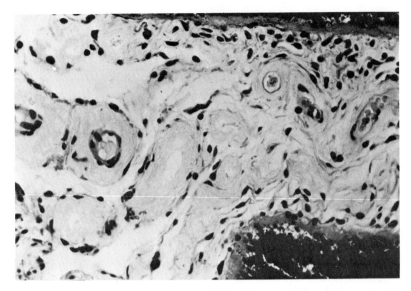

Figure 3. Photomicrograph of basal sector iridectomy specimen showing normal pigmented epithelial layers of iris. Formalin-fixed, paraffin-embedded. Hematoxylin and eosin, 500X. Marker = 50μM.

this technique. Letters describing the purpose of the study, the technique and its risks/advantages were sent on two to three occasions to patients with iridocyclitis and a comparable number of controls. Informed consent was obtained from patients who were then studied by the second author in the Glaucoma Consultation Service of the Massachusetts Eye & Ear Infirmary.

Color photographs of both eyes were taken at 16X and 25X with a Zeiss photo slit-lamp and Kodak Hi Speed Ektachrome film. Fluorescein angiograms were then taken on the same apparatus fitted with paired synchronous motor-driven cameras to provide a stereoscopic record. An intravenous injection of 10% sodium fluorescein 2 to 5cc (depending on weight of patient) was made as a bolus into an antecubital vein. Rapid sequence photographs (every two to three seconds) were then made of the dye transit in the affected eye. The light source was a Xenon flash-lamp fitted with an appropriate exciting filter and photographs were recorded on Kodak Tri-X film through matched blocking filters in each camera. Later in the sequence intermittent photographs of the opposite eye were taken for comparison.

Of 15 patients suitable for the study, seven agreed to participate; two had no ocular abnormalities, five had iridocyclitis, usually quiescent at the time of the study. Brief case summaries are presented below.

Case 1. E.D. was a 15-year-old female with oligoarticular JRA but no history of iridocyclitis. Her ocular examination was completely normal at the time of the angiogram. Angiogram result: normal study OU.

Case 2. L.M. was a 10-year-old female with monoarticular JRA and iritis intermittently active since 1974; at the time of the iris angiogram only a trace flare was present OD, no cells were seen OS. Abnormal ocular findings had included posterior synechiae present in 1974 which broke with intensive mydriasis, pigment clumps on the anterior lens plus incipient posterior subcapsular cataract. Angiogram results: normal study OU.

Case 3. M.S. was a 14-year-old male with polyarticular JRA and iritis OS at the time of iris angiography, which, however, revealed no abnormalities. He also had psoriasis.

Case 4. I.G. was a 31-year-old female with polyarticular JRA and no history of iridocyclitis. Her only ocular abnormality was gold deposition in the corneal stroma. The angiogram showed spotty fluorescein leakage at the pupillary margin apparently not associated with vascular proliferation.

Case 5. P.L. was a seven and one-half-year-old female with monoarticular JRA and iridocyclitis since age four and one-half with intermittent activity for three years on treatment. At the time of the angiogram there was trace flare OS but no inflammatory cells. Except for slight anisocoria the ocular examination was normal. The angiogram revealed abnormal leakage of capillaries at the pupillary margin OS.

Case 6. P.D. was a 19-year-old male with monarticular JRA and recurrent iritis OS for six to seven years. At the time of the angiogram there was low grade inflammation OS. Ocular abnormalities included posterior synechiae, an early cataract, and very slight band keratopathy. Angiography results: OD normal (no history of iridocyclitis in this eye); OS had leakage from the iris at the pupil with areas of delayed filling and neovascularization of the iris face. There was also prominent leakage of dye from the posterior chamber OS.

Case 7. A.P. was a 24-year-old female with monoarticular JRA. Ocular examinations were normal until age 19 when she developed acute iridocyclitis OD. Later she developed papillitis/papilledema with cystoid macular edema all of which cleared with intensive steroid treatment. There were no pupillary abnormalities. She had active iridocyclitis OD at the time of the angiogram, which revealed extensive fluorescein leakage OD from a fine network of abnormal vessels covering a major portion of the iris and fine capillaries at the pupil OS which are also probably abnormal although no definite leakage is seen.

The most common abnormality in this group of patients was leakage of dye at the pupillary margin found in three of the five patients with a history of iritis. Leakage at this site is frequently found in conditions known to be associated with abnormalities of the iris circulation such as diabetes and occlusion of the central retinal vein[12,13] and may be found in 30% of healthy eyes in patients over 50.[14] The finding is not, therefore, specific for JRA though it represents a definite abnormality in these young patients and demonstrates the ability of the angiogram to reveal pathologic changes despite clinical appearance of a "quiet eye."

Even more striking was the neovascularization on the anterior iris surface in two patients, A.P. and P.D. (Figures 4-A, 4-B, 4-C, and 4-D). Here again a pathologic change quite evident on angiogram was not detectable even on careful retrospective clinical examination; only a somewhat flattened smoother iris topography could be seen on comparison with the patients' normal eye.

Furthermore the open fish net patterns of new surface vessels especially evident in patient A.P., appears distinct from the more tightly packed convolutions of new vessels predominating near the pupil in diabetic neovascularization. This suggests that the pattern of new vessel growth may reflect to some degree the underlying disease, a situation which would carry both diagnostic and investigational importance. The significance of this neovascular pattern in JRA awaits more extensive studies.

Another interesting finding was a notable entrance of fluorescein through the pupil from the posterior chamber in patient P.D. This clearly points to excess leakage of fluorescein into the posterior aqueous humor and implicates the ciliary body in the inflammatory process.

Thus fluorescein angiography has revealed in a dramatic way, that neovascularization of the iris occurs in JRA iridocyclitis. The vessels were not visible with slit-lamp biomicroscopy but their presence undoubtedly accounts in part, for the altered iris surface texture and for the persistent aqueous humor flare seen so often in advanced cases. However, it should be noted that leakage of fluorescein is not necessarily a marker for leakage of protein since the dye is only incompletely bound to serum protein; and therefore the source of protein flare cannot be definitively determined by this technique. Still, any site leaking protein should reasonably leak fluorescein as well, so these studies can help to select the possible points of protein leakage.

The stimulus to vascular leakage and new vessel growth may be persistent inflammation. Experimental data have shown that antigen-antibody complexes may pass a leaky blood-aqueous barrier[15,16] and after complement fixation, cause an inflammatory reaction. Possibly the eye is responding to immune complexes formed elsewhere in the body.

Fluorescein angiography adds a new level of information to our study of JRA patients by revealing functional and morphologic abnormalities of the anterior segment circulation not otherwise obtainable. This may lead to a fuller understanding of the disease and help to

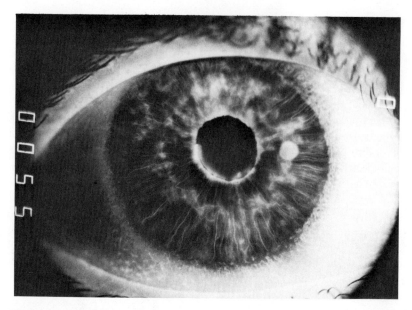

Figure 4A. Early phase angiogram in patient A.P. shows loose pattern of new vessels on iris surface with early leakage beginning superiorly. Also leakage from the pupillary margin.

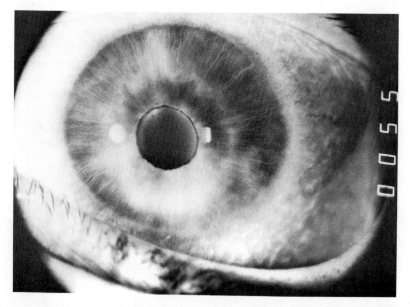

Figure 4B. Later phase of Figure A shows diffuse leakage from neovascularization.

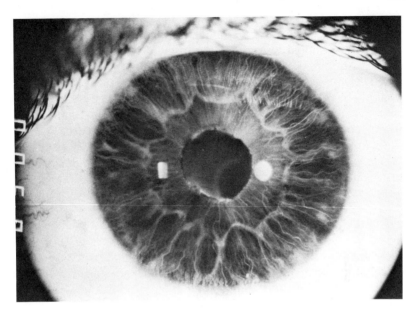

Figure 4C. Patient P.D. shows leakage at pupil from irregular patch of new vessels. Note front of fluorescein dye in pupil which originated in posterior chamber and which suggests inflammation of ciliary body.

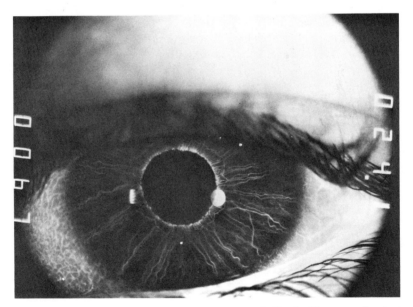

Figure 4D. Patient P.L. demonstrates most common finding in this group of patients: leakage at pupillary margin without other abnormality.

identify patients at risk for developing some of the more severe complications of JRA iritis. This technique is not applicable to very young patients but it should be useful in the study of severe inflammation and glaucoma reported to be a problem by some authors.[3] Certainly repeated fluorescein angiography of patients with neovascularization should help to clarify the risk that new vessel formation presents to these eyes. Iris angiography in as many JRA patients with iridocyclitis as possible might indicate if the leaking vessels precede or follow active inflammation. If they precede inflammation, possibly immune complexes formed elsewhere in the body are eliciting the inflammatory response.

PATTERNS OF PATIENT CARE

Questionnaires were mailed to 28 rheumatologists and 20 ophthalmologists working in 23 different American and Canadian medical centers with the purpose of detecting strengths, weaknesses, and potentially significant differences among the various centers delivering care to JRA patients. All rheumatologists responding to the questionnaire were university-affiliated physicians. Thirty-eight percent expressed dissatisfaction with arrangements made to provide their patients with ophthalmologic care principally because of frequent turnover of ophthalmic staff (i.e., residents or young staff rotating through a JRA program but establishing no long-term affiliation with patients or other staff). The average length of affiliation of an ophthalmologist with a JRA group was two years. In 75% of the cases no single rheumatologist was responsible for reviewing ocular progress of JRA patients; also 75% of responding rheumatologists indicated that ophthalmologists had not been invited to review the ocular progress of their JRA patients or present their therapeutic results for discussion. Rheumatologists frequently took responsibility for explaining the nature of the ocular disease and the risks of treatment to parents and patients, and arranged for ophthalmic care in the home community, if necessary.

Very little clinical or laboratory research is directly related to the ocular problems of JRA. In only three of 23 centers was JRA research directly related to the ocular manifestations. Only six centers reported publishing their ophthalmic experience.

The dissatisfaction expressed by the rheumatologists was felt also by ophthalmologists responding to the questionnaire, who mentioned the remoteness of their collaboration with other members of the JRA team as a significant problem and indicated that in 16 of 20 cases their responsibilities were exclusively in the area of clinical care. Only four ophthalmologists were involved in clinical or basic research on JRA. Seventy percent of ophthalmologists followed no organized examination protocol. It was surprising that 14 of 20 did not indicate an awareness that the pauciarticular JRA patient had a significantly higher risk of ocular involvement and therefore needed more frequent exams.

Treatment of iridocyclitis varied little among the ophthalmologists, practically all relying on topical and/or systemic corticosteroids and topical mydriatics; only one using immunosuppressives. Three indicated they used mydriatic-cycloplegic drugs only if posterior synechiae were present, a peculiar rationale since these drugs usually do not break established posterior synechiae, their use being to prevent synechiae formation.

In spite of Praeger's[15] and L.T. Chylack's (unpublished experience) success with phacoemulsification for cataract extraction in this population, many ophthalmologists expressed pessimism about surgical treatment of these complicated cataracts. Glaucoma surgery was regarded as quite unsuccessful while treatment of band keratopathy was successful but usually short-lived. Ophthalmologists manifested ambivalence and frustration with rheumatologists for "over-referring too many normals" while at the same time mentioning that rheumatologists do not always realize that a "white and quiet" eye may harbor significant inflammation. They were also concerned with their inability to estimate the risk of cataract from continuing low-grade inflammation vs chronic steroid use. In spite of these problems over 90% of ophthalmologists planned to continue their affiliation with a JRA program.

At the Robert Breck Brigham Hospital the following general guidelines are used in managing ophthalmologic problems in patients with JRA:

1. All patients with presumed or diagnosed JRA have a full ocular examination (including slit-lamp biomicroscopy) at the time of initial visit.
2. Those with diagnosed pauciarticular JRA are examined every three to four months until late adolescence, when, if they have been free of ocular disease, the frequency of examinations is reduced.
3. Those with polyarticular disease are seen every six to 12 months.
4. Those with active or inactive iridocyclitis, regardless of the type of arthritis are seen every three months or as frequently as necessary.

5. The medical treatment follows the scheme shown in Table 1.

6. When aqueous humor is free of cells the dose of topical and/or systemic corticosteroid is gradually reduced. The patient is always reexamined a few days after steroids are discontinued to look for recurrent disease.

7. Persistent aqueous flare is not a sufficient reason for continuing topical steroid therapy.

8. Mydriatic/cycloplegics are always the last drugs to be stopped.

The patterns of patient care which emerged from the survey suggest that closer collaboration between ophthalmologist and rheumatologist would eliminate many of the communication gaps which hinder efforts to provide the best care. Only through cooperation among several centers can such questions as the relative risk of cataract from low-grade iridocyclitis or chronic steroids be assessed. Ophthalmologists who are interested enough in these patients to collaborate for several years could make a more thorough review of national or worldwide experience with ocular manifestations of JRA.

SPECULATIONS

Incidence

JRA patients who develop iridocyclitis are usually seronegative for rheumatoid factor.[17] However, the quantitative antinuclear antibody (ANA) test has been useful in estimating the risk of developing iridocyclitis.[18] In one study by Stillman et al. 52% of patients with iridocyclitis had ANA as opposed to 35% without. When quantitative titers were measured 31% of patients with iridocylitis had ANA titers

Table 1

The scheme of medical treatment of iridocyclitis at the Robert Breck Brigham Hospital

Drug	State of Iridocyclitis		
	Mild	Moderate	Severe
Phenylephrine 10%	+	±	±
Atropine or scopolamine		+	+
Prednisolone acetate drops	+		±
Decadron ophthalmic ointment		+	+
Sub-Tenon's Depo-Medrol			±
Systemic steroids			±

of 1/160 or more as compared to only 9% of patients without eye disease.[18]

The method of calculating relative risk has been published by Gibson et al.[19]

$$x = \frac{hK}{Hk}$$

x = relative risk
h = % of patients with a particular marker
k = % of patients not having a particular marker
H = % of controls with particular marker
K = % of controls without particular marker

If Stillman's data are used in this formula, the risk of the disease for a female with pauciarticular arthritis and an ANA titer of 1/20 or more, and the onset of JRA before two years of age is 95.7%.[18] In contrast, females with systemic onset or polyarticular onset JRA with similar characteristics had risks of 77.9% and 84.7% respectively. The combination of parameters of age, sex, type of onset of arthritis, and antinuclear antibody titer allows definition of groups at greatest risk of developing iridocyclitis.

Genetics

Of extreme importance is the clarification of the prevalence of HLA antigens in JRA (see Chapter 8). If man is shown to have distinct immune-response genes similar to the H-2 major histocompatibility complex in the mouse, there may be a genetic explanation for the disposition of some JRA patients to have severe blinding iridocyclitis and others to be free of ocular involvement. Certainly to date there has been no correlation between HLA antigens and iridocyclitis.

The prevalence of HLA-B27 antigen in juvenile rheumatoid arthritis is controversial. As correctly emphasized by Gibson et al. a conservative approach to statistical analysis of the significance of B27 antigen should be employed until sufficiently long-term data are gathered from groups of patients who clearly meet the criteria for JRA.[19] These studies will favor detection of ankylosing spondylitis and allow the omission of these cases from the study.

SUMMARY

Iris specimens obtained at cataract surgery were studied anatomically. All eyes were free of active iridocyclitis at the time of surgery. There were very few abnormalities seen; of possible significance is a slight round-cell infiltrate along the anterior iris border and possibly a slight increase in the number of iris vessels. No superficial iris neovascularization was found.

Patients meeting the criteria for juvenile rheumatoid arthritis were studied with fluorescein iris angiography. Abnormal leakage from pupillary vessels was found in several cases of mild iridocyclitis; in advanced iridocyclitis, there were areas of delayed filling and extensive neovascularization of the iris face, from which fluorescein leakage occurred. Leakage originating in the posterior chamber suggested a possible abnormality in the ciliary body.

A survey of the patterns of care by rheumatologists and ophthalmologists collaborating to provide care to JRA patients and their families is discussed.

Recent immunologic and genetic advances are also discussed along with some significant problems in the management of JRA.

REFERENCES

1. Calabro, J.J., Holgerson, W.B., Sonpol, G.M., and Khoury, M.I. Juvenile rheumatoid arthritis: a general review and report of 100 patients observed for 15 years. *Semin Arthritis Rheum.* 5:257–98, 1976.

2. Spalter, H.F. The visual prognosis in juvenile rheumatoid arthritis. *Trans Am Ophthalmol Soc.* 72:554–70, 1975.

3. Key, S.N., III, and Kimura, S.I. Iridocyclitis associated with juvenile rheumatoid arthritis. *Am J Ophthalmol.* 80:425–9, 1975.

4. Chylack, L.T., Jr., Bienfang, D.C., Bellows, A.R., and Stillman, J.S. Ocular manifestations of juvenile rheumatoid arthritis. *Am J Ophthalmol.* 79:1026–33, 1975.

5. Chylack, L.T., Jr. Ocular manifestations of juvenile rheumatoid arthritis. Experience with 210 cases. *Arthritis Rheum.* 20 (suppl):217–23, 1977.

6. Stewart, A.J., and Hill, R.H. Ocular manifestations in juvenile rheumatoid arthritis. *Can J Ophthalmol.* 2:58, 1967.

7. Smiley, W.K., May, E., and Bywaters, E.G.L. Ocular presentations in Still's disease and their treatment. *Ann Rheum Dis.* 16:371, 1957.

8. Smiley, W.K. Iridocyclitis in Still's disease. *Trans Ophthalmol Soc UK.* 85:351, 1965.

9. Smiley, W.K. The eye in juvenile rheumatoid arthritis. *Trans Ophthalmol Soc UK.* 94:817–29, 1964.

10. Brewer, E.J., Jr., Bass, J.C., Cassidy, J.T. et al. Criteria for the classification of juvenile rheumatoid arthritis. *Bull Rheum Dis.* 23:712–19, 1973.

11. Muller, L.L., and Jacks, T.J. Rapid chemical dehydration of samples for electron microscopic examination. *J Histochem Cytochem.* 23:107–10, 1975.

12. Jensen, V.A., and Lundboek, K. Fluorescence angiography of the iris in recent and long-term diabetes. *Acta Ophthalmol.* 46:584, 1968.

13. Raitta, C., and Vannas, S. Fluoresceinangiographie der Irisgefasse nach Zentralvenen verschluss. *Graefes Arch klin exp Ophthal.* 177 (1):33–8, 1969.

14. Vannas, A. Fluorescein angiography of the vessels of the iris in pseudoexfoliation of the lens capsule, capsular glaucoma, and some other forms of glaucoma. *Acta Ophthalmol.* (suppl) 105, 1969.

15. Praeger, D.L., Schneider, H.A., Sakowski, A.D., Jr., and Jacobs, J.C. Kelman procedure in the treatment of complicated cataract of the uveitis of Still's disease. *Trans Ophthalmol Soc UK.* 96:168–72, 1976.

16. Wong, V.G., Anderson, R.R., and McMaster, P.R. Endogenous immune uveitis. *Arch Ophthalmol.* 85:93–102, 1971.

17. Kanski, J.J. Clinical and immunological study of anterior uveitis in juvenile rheumatoid arthritis. *Trans Ophthalmol Soc UK.* 96:123–30, 1976.

18. Stillman, J.S., Barry, P.E., and Bell, C.L. Clinical characteristics and classification of juvenile rheumatoid arthritis. Symposium in Bristol, England, January 1975.

19. Gibson, D.J., Carpenter, C.B., Stillman, J.S., and Schur, P.H. Histocompatibility antigens in patients with juvenile rheumatoid arthritis. *N Engl J Med.* 293:636–8, 1975.

13 Carditis in JRA

John J. Miller III

Pericarditis is uniformly recognized as a feature of systemic juvenile rheumatoid arthritis (JRA). However, data regarding incidence and opinions regarding clinical significance vary at different centers. While I am convinced that myocarditis is a rare but distinct complication of JRA, this remains a controversial point of view. Nevertheless, the treatment of all cardiac manifestations of JRA is straightforward and generally agreed upon.

PERICARDITIS

Incidence

The classical description of pericarditis in JRA is that of Lietman and Bywaters who described 20 cases of clinical pericarditis which had been recognized among 285 children with JRA, an incidence of seven percent.[1] All the children had elevated sedimentation rates. The other manifestations of systemic disease were far more common in these children than in ones in whom pericarditis was not recognized. More importantly however, was that five of 11 autopsies of JRA patients revealed pericardial disease, and only one of the five had been diagnosed as having clinical pericarditis. The authors concluded that pericarditis occurred more frequently than diagnosed, but that when subclinical it was benign.

The advent of echocardiography should have provided a painless noninvasive way of confirming this idea. Bernstein, Takahashi and Hanson[2] reported an echocardiographic study in which 55% of 29 patients with systemic mode of onset, 33% of 12 patients with polyarticular onset, and none of 14 patients with pauciarticular onset had pericardial effusions. Only four of the patients had had friction rubs, eight had abnormal ECGs and nine had increased cardiac size by radiography. None of 38 normal children had evidence of pericardial effusions by the same echocardiographic criteria. In contrast, Brewer found effusions by echocardiography in only five of 50 consecutive patients, and three of the five had symptoms of pericarditis.[3] He concluded asymptomatic pericarditis was not common.

The difference in these two studies was probably due to a greater proportion of patients with systemic mode of onset in Bernstein et al.'s group.[2] However, artifacts may cause errors in reading echocardiographs and not all criteria for diagnosis of effusions are rigid. The apparent low incidence found by Brewer is not inconsistent with the autopsy data since pericarditis may be episodic, and fibrous adhesions reported by Lietman and Bywater[1] may have resulted from transient rather than chronically persisting disease.

It is safe to say only that subclinical pericarditis occurs in JRA, and that both subclinical and clinically significant pericardial effusions are most frequent in children with active systemic disease.

Diagnosis and Course

Clinically significant pericarditis will be associated with physical signs or symptoms such as sharp precordial pain which changes with respiration or position, and dyspnea.[1,3,4] Tachycardia, tachypnea, pallor, muffled heart sounds, and friction rub are the signs in mild to moderately severe cases.[1,3,4] Severe cases are unusual but may progress to tamponade and failure, with distended neck veins and hepatomegaly.[3,4]

The most sensitive method for making the diagnosis of pericarditis, echocardiography, is not yet a practical screening procedure for most clinics. Electrocardiograms have typical but not dramatic abnormalities. Lietman and Bywaters described T-wave inversion and ST-segment elevation.[1] McNamara and Brewer[4] provide a much more detailed description of the significance of T-wave changes and point out that ST-segment shifts must be balanced so that both elevated and depressed segments are seen. PR intervals are normal. Chest radiographs may show a large, globular cardiac shape.[1,3,4]

Lietman and Bywaters felt that the pericarditis of JRA had a benign and self-limited course. The longest duration of effusion they observed was 14 weeks, although intermittent recurrent courses were seen. However, Brewer has described two of 20 patients with cardiac disease who developed tamponade with congestive failure, one having had persistent effusion for 11 years. Constrictive pericarditis has not yet been reported in children. Death due to pericarditis must be very rare considering a review of 130 deaths of children with JRA from 21 centers in Europe, the Pacific and the United States which revealed that less than 10% of deaths were from heart disease and that half of these were due to amyloidosis.[5]

Treatment

Most children with pericarditis of JRA could probably do quite well if observed carefully and treated with adequate levels of salicylates. However, it becomes difficult to maintain a conservative approach when viewing the sometimes dramatic temperature and pulse graphs and chest radiographs. Lietman and Bywaters did not believe adrenocorticosteroids were effective, but this is not the current opinion.[1,3,4] Indeed, Calabro suggests the early use of steroids when symptomatic pericarditis is present because of the possibility of underlying myocarditis which might leave permanent damage (see below).[6] The moment at which steroids are added to salicylate therapy will vary with each physician's ability to handle his own anxiety, but clear criteria are (1) persistent or recurring chest pain, (2) dyspnea, or (3) signs of impending tamponade or congestive heart failure. Prednisone in doses of 60 mg/M^2/day in single or divided doses will be effective for most patients although a few may require intravenous hydrocortisone in doses up to 500 mg every six hours. Response is usually very rapid but weaning from steroids is often associated with flaring disease. Pericardiocentesis may be required, and appropriate instruments should be available and appropriate personnel alerted when a patient with symptomatic pericarditis is admitted to hospital, whether a decision is made to use steroids or not.

MYOCARDITIS

Incidence

Some pediatric rheumatologists doubt that clinically significant myocarditis exists as part of JRA. However, two reports have appeared from different centers describing a consistent clinical picture of congestive heart failure occurring in the absence of extracardiac cause and leaving a hypertrophied myocardium.[8,9] Some believe such episodes are due to coincidental viral myocarditis, and this is impossible to disprove completely. However, the cases seen at Stanford have not had identifiable antiviral antibodies, and three of our four patients have had recurrent episodes.[9,11] These four children were seen between 1965 and 1977 during which time about 400 cases of JRA were seen at Stanford. Good, Venters, Page and Good saw one case of myocarditis in 150 consecutive patients with JRA, but do not provide a description of the clinical picture other than indicating presence of congestive heart failure.[10] Jordan has reported the highest incidence of myocarditis, three in 30 cases of JRA, but all of these patients had been referred specifically to a cardiac clinic, so the data are not representative for all JRA patients.[8] Bernstein et al. described prolonged systolic ejection times in two of 40 and prolonged preejection times in four of 40 patients with JRA, and suggested that this was evidence of myocarditis, however, none of these patients had clinical cardiac disease.

Diagnosis and Course

The diagnosis is entirely an operational one: the child develops congestive heart failure in the absence of significant pericardial effusion, hypertension, valve abnormality, or extracardiac cause. This occurs on a background of active systemic disease and is heralded by a persisting tachycardia which does not rise and fall consistently with the usual spiking fevers. ECGs are not distinguishable from those seen in pericarditis, but premature ventricular contractions and conduction abnormalities may develop, Figure 1. Chest radiographs may or may not show cardiomegaly but if they do it will be out of proportion to the amount of pericardial fluid present, Figure 2. Echocardiograms show dilated ventricles and an increase in ventricle wall thickness, particularly after repeated episodes. Myocardial hypertrophy has persisted by ECG criteria, chest radiography, and echocardiography in three of the four patients seen at Stanford. Two of these children have died, but both died of complications of drug therapy, not from heart disease.[9,11]

There are no reports of acute pathology. The heart of a child who died two years after her last episode of carditis had dilated ventricles, thickened walls and a fine, diffuse interstitial fibrosis.[11] One other child died two months after an acute episode while still receiving high doses of prednisone.[9] His heart also had dilated ventricles, and thickened walls with mild but distinct interstitial infiltrate of lymphocytes and polymorphonuclear cells, Figure 3. Muscle fibers and nuclei were markedly and paradoxically varied in size, Figure 4. This proves that a myocardial disease had been present, but does not distinguish the exact process.[12]

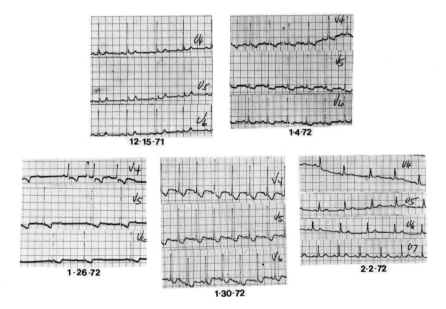

Figure 1. Recordings of ECG leads V_4 through V_6 from boy at varied stages of episode of myocarditis. Dec. 15, 1971: clinically well but receiving digoxin 0.010 mg/kg/day. Jan. 4, 1972: tachycardia, depressed ST-segments and inverted T-waves, not in congestive heart failure. Pattern consistent with isolated pericarditis. Three weeks later: full flare of disease, developed second-degree heart block with Wenckebach phenomenon. No change in digoxin dose. Digoxin stopped, intravenous hydrocortisone given with rapid clinical improvement and return to a normal ECG in one week.

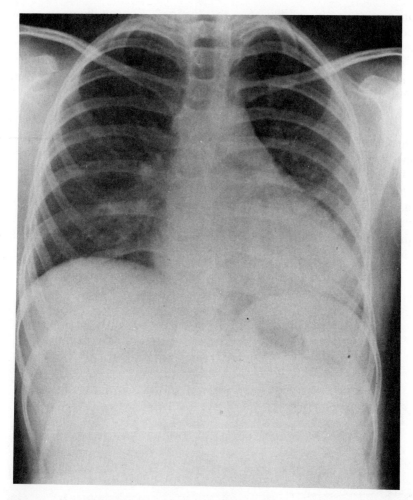

Figure 2. Chest radiograph of a girl following episode of myocarditis. Despite enlarged and globular cardiac shadow, no pericardial fluid seen by echocardiography at this time. Subsequent decrease in size, but after repeated episodes patient has constantly enlarged heart.

Treatment

In my experience, acute episodes thought to be myocarditis have always responded within 24 or 48 hours to treatment with adrenocorticosteroids and diuretics. Hydrocortisone, 100–500 mg intravenously every four to six hours is followed by 60 mg/M²/day prednisone orally. Different diuretics have been used without problems, and the diuretic

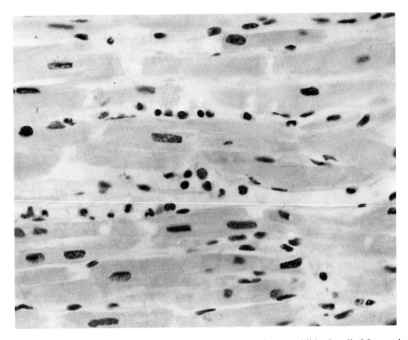

Figure 3. Photomicrograph of section of myocardium from a child who died 2 months after acute episode of carditis. Mild but distinct interstitial infiltrate of polymorphonuclear cells and lymphocytes despite fact that high doses of adrenocorticosteroids have had to be maintained to prevent recurrent tachycardia. H&E. × 500.

of choice is probably the one with which the physician is most familiar. Three of our four patients have been digitalized but two have developed toxicity even at low doses.[9] Digitalis should therefore be avoided if possible. The greatest problems occur during the weaning from steroids as these patients will flare with renewed tachycardia or arrhythmias when the drugs are reduced too rapidly or too far. Two of the children followed at Stanford have appeared to respond to gold therapy, allowing complete steroid withdrawal, while the other two required almost constant maintenance doses of prednisone.[9,11]

SUMMARY

The incidence of pericarditis and of myocarditis in JRA is still unknown. Indeed, even the existence of the latter is questioned by some. Probably both are infrequent yet still occur more frequently than diagnosed. Salicylates and observation are therapy enough for most cases of pericarditis, but some will require pericardiocentesis. Pericar-

172

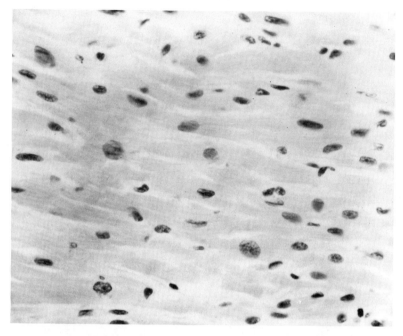

Figure 4. Photomicrograph of another area of myocardium from same case shown Figure 3. Fibers and nuclei vary greatly in size. Large nuclei present in some small fibers, evidence of past hypertrophy and of certain but undefined myocardial disease. H&E. × 500.

ditis and myocarditis respond rapidly to adrenocorticosteroids, and these should be used if tamponade or congestive heart failure appear imminent.

REFERENCES

1. Lietman, P.S., and Bywaters, E.G.L. Pericarditis in juvenile rheumatoid arthritis. *Pediatrics.* 32:855–60, 1963.
2. Bernstein, B., Takahashi, M., and Hanson, V. Cardiac involvement in juvenile rheumatoid arthritis. *J Pediatr.* 85:313–17, 1974.
3. Brewer, E., Jr. Juvenile rheumatoid arthritis-cardiac involvement. *Arthritis Rheum.* 20 (suppl):231–6, 1977.
4. McNamara, D.G., and Brewer, E., Jr. Carditis with rheumatoid arthritis. Edited by E.J. Brewer, Jr. In *Juvenile Rheumatoid Arthritis.* Philadelphia: W.B. Saunders Co., 1970.
5. Baum, J., and Gutowska, G. Death in juvenile rheumatoid arthritis. *Arthritis Rheum.* 20 (suppl):253–5, 1977.
6. Calabro, J.J. Management of juvenile rheumatoid arthritis. *J Pediatr.* 77:355–65, 1970.

7. West, R.J. Acute polyarthritis: diagnosis and management. Edited by B. Ansell. In *Clinics in Rheumatic Diseases,* Vol. 2. London: W.B. Saunders Co., Ltd., 1976, pp. 305–37.

8. Jordan, J.D. Cardiopulmonary manifestations of rheumatoid disease in childhood. *South Med J.* 57:1273–7, 1964.

9. Miller, J.J., III, and French, J.W. Myocarditis in juvenile rheumatoid arthritis. *Am J Dis Child.* 131:205–9, 1977.

10. Good, R.A., Venters, H., Page, A.R., and Good, T.A. Diffuse connective tissue diseases in childhood. *Journal Lancet* 81:192–204, 1961.

11. Miller, J.J., III, Williams, G.F., and Leissring, J.C. Multiple late complications of therapy with cyclophosphamide, including ovarian destruction. *Am J Med.* 50:530–5, 1971.

12. Roberts, W.C., and Ferrans, V.J. The pathologic anatomy of the cardiomyopathies. *Hum Pathol.* 6:287–342, 1975.

14 Medical Therapy of Juvenile Rheumatoid Arthritis

Bram H. Bernstein
Donald M. Thompson
Bernhard H. Singsen

Drug therapy of juvenile rheumatoid arthritis (JRA) is complex because of the lack of controlled studies on the efficacy and toxicity of most medications in common use, resultant reliance on studies performed in adult rheumatoid arthritis (RA), incomplete understanding of mechanisms of action and, in some cases, the proscription of certain drugs for certain age groups because of adverse case reports. More recently, a welcome change in FDA policy has limited marketing of new antirheumatic medications until testing in children has been completed. While this policy slows the addition of new therapies it increases our understanding of these drugs as they become available, and has encouraged development of multicenter collaborative study techniques in pediatric rheumatology.

In this chapter medications are presented according to their mechanisms of action as currently understood. The rapid-acting antiinflammatory drugs including aspirin, nonsteroidal antiinflammatory drugs (NSAID), and indomethacin, appear to operate at least in part by inhibiting synthesis of the prostaglandins. The slower-acting

175

antiinflammatory drugs including gold, hydroxychloroquine, and d-penicillamine, may alter the functioning of phagocytic cells (neutrophils and macrophages). Corticosteroids while the most potent antiinflammatory agents, are dealt with subsequently to emphasize their tertiary role in the treatment of JRA. In contrast immunosuppressive agents may alter the pathogenesis of JRA at an earlier stage, but remain an experimental mode of therapy at this time.

Each child with JRA presents a unique challenge to medical therapy techniques, and thus an individualized and flexible approach to treatment must always be maintained.

ASPIRIN

Aspirin has been used in the treatment of both adult rheumatoid arthritis (RA) and JRA since the beginning of the twentieth century.[1] In spite of the tremendous amount of experience with aspirin, unanswered questions regarding the mechanism of its antiinflammatory effect remain. Nevertheless, knowledge concerning the mode of action and potential toxic effects of aspirin has increased greatly, and it continues to be the drug of choice for initial therapy of JRA because of its efficacy in most patients, its relative safety when properly used, and its low cost.

Aspirin is most rapidly absorbed as the intact, nonionized, lipid-soluble molecule from the stomach and upper GI tract by passive diffusion through the gastric mucosa and underlying cells.[2] At the usual pH of gastric juice the salicylate molecule is predominantly in nonionized form. If the pH of the stomach is increased the aspirin molecule becomes ionized and is less rapidly absorbed. However, overall rate of absorption may not be reduced since solubility is enhanced at higher pH, and dissolution of the aspirin tablet is therefore more rapid.[3]

Following absorption, the acetylsalicylic acid molecule is rapidly hydrolyzed to salicylic acid in plasma, liver, and red blood cells. Fifty to eighty percent of serum salicylate is bound to plasma protein; this is important as there is evidence that it is only nonbound salicylate molecule which is active. This binding is reversible.[2] The concentration of salicylate in the blood is therefore related to the level of plasma proteins, particularly albumin. It follows that patients with active JRA who frequently have low serum albumin will have lower concentrations of protein-bound salicylate, and lower serum salicylate levels.

Salicylate is excreted primarily by the kidney. Under conditions of normal renal function and urinary pH, only ten percent is excreted as free salicylic acid, and the remainder as salicylic acid conjugates which are formed in the liver, and whose excretion is little influenced by urinary pH. In alkaline urine up to 85% of salicylate may be excreted as free salicylic acid, whereas in acid urine, only 10% is excreted in this form.[2] Efforts to reduce renal excretion of aspirin and thus increase serum salicylate levels by further acidifying the urine are generally unsuccessful; further acidification of urine already at a pH of six or below achieves little change in the degree of retention of free salicylic acid.[4]

The exact mechanism by which salicylates exert their antiinflammatory effect is still not fully undertstood. Aspirin produces a reduction in lymphocyte blastogenesis in vitro, but in vivo studies show little evidence of it having an immunosuppressive effect.[5,6] In recent years studies have suggested that prostaglandins may be important mediators of inflammation by virtue of their effects upon blood vessels, and aspirin has been shown to produce inhibition of prostaglandin synthetase.[7,8] Whatever its mechanism of action, aspirin undoubtedly exerts an antiinflammatory effect in dosages sufficient to produce serum salicylate levels around 25 mg%.

Our practice is to begin all new JRA patients, with the exception of those known to be allergic to salicylates, on an aspirin dose of 80/mg/kg/day or less in four divided doses. After a period of three to seven days, serum salicylate and transaminase levels are checked. If the patient's response has been less than optimal, i.e., the salicylate level less than 20 to 25 mg%, and transaminase levels are normal, aspirin dosage is increased. Small increments in aspirin dosage may lead to large increments in serum salicylate levels so aspirin doses should be increased slowly and cautiously.[9] Since the half-life of salicylate is prolonged at higher serum levels four divided doses are generally adequate and children need not be awakened for aspirin at night.[9] Patients receiving concomitant steroid therapy should be observed for increasing serum salicylate levels and clinical signs of aspirin toxicity during steroid reduction. This is necessary because steroids alter the renal clearance of aspirin. As steroids are withdrawn aspirin excretion decreases and serum salicylate levels may increase,[10] so therapy is continued until there have been no signs of clinically active disease for several months, after which it is gradually withdrawn.

This relatively conservative use of aspirin reflects the recent recognition of a high incidence of aspirin-induced hepatotoxicity in JRA patients, and the development of frank salicylism in some of our younger patients treated with the heretofore standard dosage of 100 mg/kg/day.[11,12] The hepatotoxicity due to aspirin is dose-dependent, but there is great individual variation in sensitivity so some children develop elevated transaminase levels on relatively low doses, whereas others can tolerate much larger amounts. Vague abdominal discomfort, anorexia, and sometimes vomiting are common with transaminase levels over 100 IU. While generally mild and reversible when aspirin dose is reduced or discontinued, very high transaminase elevations (over 1000 IU/L) have occurred, and children suffering from even mild dehydration due to intercurrent infections seem more likely to develop such high levels. A recent chart review of our JRA patients who have expired suggested to us that hepatotoxicity due to aspirin alone or in combination with other factors, might have contributed to these deaths. Our current practice, therefore, is to monitor transaminase levels frequently while dosages of aspirin are being adjusted, and at longer intervals in patients on constant aspirin doses. It should also be noted that doses based on body weight are often not suitable for teenagers who may develop salicylism on the standard 80–100 mg/kg/day of aspirin.

Other toxic effects of aspirin are well known. The most frequent side effect in adults is gastritis and/or peptic ulcer. In our experience children appear to be less suceptible to this; in fact, the abdominal pain in some aspirin-treated children previously thought to be due to gastric irritation may actually have represented symptoms of hepatotoxicity. Nevertheless we generally administer aspirin with food or antacid, and many patients are placed on Ascriptin rather than plain aspirin. Enteric-coated aspirin is frequently used in some centers but we have found its absorption from the GI tract to be unreliable and therefore use it infrequently.

The well known prolonged bleeding time in aspirin-treated patients due to reduced platelet aggregation and to some degree, the prolongation of prothrombin time, leads us to stop aspirin routinely one to two weeks prior to elective surgery.[13] Excessive bleeding from the minor accidents which are so common among children has not been a problem although increased bruising is frequently apparent.

Optimal therapy with any medication, especially when administered over a prolonged period of time, demands that parents and when appropriate, children, have a full understanding of the purpose of the medication, the way it must be utilized, and its potential toxic effects. It is important that patients and their families understand that aspirin must be given in adequate dosage and on a regular basis to produce an antiinflammatory effect and that the drug must be continued even when the child does not have joint pain. However, parents should be instructed to stop aspirin if their child is at risk of dehydration from vomiting or diarrhea, particularly the young child. Many parents are concerned that long-term aspirin therapy might lead to addiction or the development of tolerance and they should be reassured on this matter realizing that when properly used and when safeguards are taken, aspirin is an effective and safe treatment of JRA.

NONSTEROIDAL ANTIINFLAMMATORY DRUGS

During the past two years a number of new nonsteroidal antiinflammatory drugs have become available for the treatment of RA, and it is expected that others will be released in the near future. The NSAIDs currently available in this country include ibuprofen (Motrin), naproxen (Naprosyn), fenoprofen calcium (Nalfon), all of which are propionic acid derivatives; and tolmetin (Tolectin) which is a pyrrole derivative, chemically related to indomethacin.

Although all of these drugs are currently available for adult use, only tolmetin has received FDA approval for use in children as of December 1977. This followed conclusion of testing in a multicenter study by the Pediatric Rheumatology Collaborative Study Group.[14] Testing by this combined center group of fenoprofen calcium as well as two newer NSAIDs, proquazone and pirprofen, is currently proceeding.

Tolmetin is 1-methyl-5-p-toluoylpyrrole-2-acetic acid. It is rapidly absorbed after oral administration with peak plasma levels present 20 minutes after administration.[15] The plasma half-life is approximately one hour and the drug and its metabolites are almost completely excreted in urine within 24 hours. It is extensively bound to plasma proteins, and in vitro studies show mutual displacement from protein binding sites for both tolmetin and salicylic acid. In spite of this competitive inhibition noted in laboratory studies clinical studies show only minor changes in the plasma levels of each drug with chronic coadministration of both. Tolmetin is believed to exert its antiinflammatory effect by inhibition of prostaglandin synthetase.[16] It has also been shown to increase plasma and extracellular fluid volumes, thus causing small decreases in the concentration of hemoglobin and red blood cell counts as well as reducing serum prostaglandin-E values.[17] Since prostaglandin-E is known to cause increased renal blood flow and increased excretion of salt and water it seems likely that this increase in extracellular fluid volume is directly related to the drug-induced PgE reduction.[18] Like aspirin, tolmetin produces prolongation of the bleeding time due to decreased platelet adhesion, but unlike aspirin this is not accompanied by consistent changes in platelet aggregation.[19]

Tolmetin was studied for a four-week open trial in 30 juvenile rheumatoid patients and a subsequent 12 week double-blind trial against aspirin in 107 JRA patients by the Pediatric Rheumatology Collaborative Study Group.[14] This study demonstrated tolmetin to have antiinflammatory and analgesic properties as effective as those of aspirin in the short-term management of JRA. Only one tolmetin-treated patient, as opposed to 6 aspirin-treated patients, required withdrawal from the study because of adverse side effects. Of particular note was the finding of a sustained decrease in liver transaminase activity in the tolmetin-treated patients, whereas aspirin-treated patients showed an average increase in serum transaminase levels. The authors concluded that tolmetin was a safe and useful new drug for treatment of JRA.

Studies done on adults have also shown tolmetin to be generally as effective as aspirin in the treatment of rheumatoid arthritis but with a lower incidence of side effects, e.g., significantly less fecal blood loss was found in tolmetin-treated patients than in those treated with aspirin.[20] Therapeutic response significantly increased when it was used in combination with gold therapy and there was no increase in the incidence or severity of adverse reactions.[21] Of interest is one study which suggested the possibility of synergism between tolmetin and acetaminophen.[22] This study was carried out after animal data had demonstrated potentiation of tolmetin by acetaminophen. An adequate therapeutic response was noted in 92% of the group treated with tolmetin and acetaminophen whereas only 73% of the group treated with tolmetin plus placebo responded.

In the authors' experience this drug has shown efficacy relatively equivalent to that of aspirin in the treatment of pauci- and polyarticular JRA. The children have tolerated it well in three or four daily dosages up to a total dose of 30 mg/kg/day. We have noted false-positive reactions by sulfasalicylic acid testing but not by the dipstick method in the urine of tolmetin-treated patients. So far it has not appeared to be as useful in children with systemic JRA, since spiking fevers have reoccurred or worsened in some cases following institution of therapy. Perhaps combination with acetaminophen might produce beneficial results in such patients.

Fenoprofen calcium is currently undergoing investigation by the Pediatric Rheumatology Study Group. Eighty percent of this propionic acid derivative is absorbed following oral administration and 90% of the absorbed drug is excreted in the urine.[23] Both fenoprofen and its major metabolite, hydroxyfenoprofen, appear in urine conjugated primarily to glucuronide. Maximal plasma levels are achieved with the first few doses and further accumulation with repeated doses is minimal.[3] As with tolmetin and other NSAIDs, the drug is largely protein-bound and aspirin therapy does lead to a small decrease in plasma fenoprofen levels which appears to have little clinical significance. Fenoprofen does not, however, reduce serum salicylate levels.[23] Efficacy studies in adults have shown antiinflammatory, analgesic, and antipyretic effects roughly equivalent to those of aspirin, but the incidence of side effects particularly gastrointestinal, is significantly lower.[24-26] Our preliminary experience with fenoprofen in JRA patients suggests that it may be an effective and well tolerated antiinflammatory agent. It also appears to be very effective in controlling the fever spikes of systemic JRA.

Neither ibuprofen nor naproxen has as yet been critically studied in childhood arthritis in the United States, and formal approval by the FDA has not been given. Ibuprofen has been reported to be equal in efficacy to indomethacin with considerable less toxicity in RA.[27] Since this was the first of the NSAIDs to be made generally available our experience with it has been most extensive. Doses up to 50 mg/kg/day have been well tolerated in children and it has been useful in all forms of JRA. The manufacturers of ibuprofen suggest that it not be used in conjunction with aspirin therapy because of potential competitive inhibition; however, clinical experience suggests that some children are benefited by combination therapy. As with other NSAIDs side effects are uncommon and generally mild. Minimal fluid retention occasionally occurs, probably related to reduced levels of prostaglandins, but there has been little gastrointestinal toxicity or elevation of serum transaminases reported.[28]

Among the NSAIDs, naproxen is unique in that it has a prolonged serum half-life of 12 to 15 hours with almost total excretion via the urine within 24 hours.[29] Because of this long half-life twice a day dosage is feasible. Naproxen is a naphthyl-propionic acid which is rapidly and completely absorbed by the oral route and extensively bound to plasma proteins. Studies utilizing naproxen dosages several times higher than the clinically effective amount showed an increase in the urinary excretion rate at the higher doses, so that progressive dosage increase did not produce corresponding increments in plasma levels. These data suggest that there is a selfregulatory mechanism which, by virtue of plasma binding-site saturation limits naproxen levels in man. Studies of the interaction of naproxen and aspirin showed a rather small decrease in peak concentration levels of either drug with coadministration[30] of both which was significant only in the case of naproxen levels being reduced by aspirin. Salicylate enhanced the renal clearance of naproxen, perhaps by its displacement from binding sites on plasma proteins. Other clinical studies showed it to be relatively nontoxic when compared to aspirin, and comparable in terms of efficacy.[31,32] Of particular interest is an investigation showing that although both aspirin and naproxen prolong the bleeding time this prolongation is considerably greater with aspirin.[33] It was felt that the two probably have different mechanisms of action on platelets, such that aspirin permanently acetylates the platelet and thereby impairs its function for the life span of the platelet; whereas platelets subjected to naproxen effect may undergo functional recovery. A significant advantage of naproxen and perhaps other NSAIDs may be that, unlike aspirin, they need not be discontinued more than three or four days prior to the time that surgical procedures are carried out.

In summary the NSAIDs appear to be relatively nontoxic and comparable to aspirin in their efficacy. Since experience with them in children is as yet limited and the potential for unforeseen side effects therefore exists, it is our feeling that these drugs must still *follow* aspirin as primary therapy for JRA. Their use should be reserved for those children in whom adequate serum salicylate levels cannot be achieved because of side effects, or where there is aspirin hypersensitivity or intolerance. Their combination with aspirin may be useful in some situations in spite of the fact that aspirin may reduce plasma NSAID concentrations.

In our experience children have differed in their response to the various NSAIDs so it seems reasonable that a trial of one be given for several weeks and, in the event of an inadequate therapeutic response, that the child be switched to an alternative NSAID. However, it has been our general impression that where aspirin in adequate dosage was clearly ineffective in controlling disease little advantage resulted from changing to NSAID therapy.

INDOMETHACIN

Indomethacin is an indole derivative (1-p-chlorobenzoyl-5-methoxy-2-methylindole-3-acetic acid) which became available for clinical trials in 1961 and for general prescribing in 1965. Initial reports of its efficacy in the rheumatic diseases were enthusiastic, but subsequent studies showed little advantage over aspirin therapy.[34-36]

The drug is easily absorbed by the oral route and peak serum levels are present at one to two hours. The plasma half-life is about one and one-half hours in healthy adults and even shorter in school-age children.[37] Indomethacin is highly protein-bound, conjugated with glucuronide in liver, and excreted in bile and urine. Two-thirds of the dose is excreted via the kidneys and one-third through the gastrointestinal tract.[38] Standard criteria for antiinflammatory effect in animals show it to be potent and also to have antipyretic and analgesic properties.[38] It appears to be a powerful inhibitor of prostaglandin biosynthesis, many times more so than aspirin on a milligram-for-milligram basis.[39] Unfortunately, side effects of indomethacin are relatively frequent, the major ones being headache and gastric upset. More serious but less common side effects have included severe depression, dizziness, rare psychotic reactions, as well as GI bleeding, ulceration, and perforation.[40] Corneal deposits or retinal lesions have rarely been noted;[41] reports of leukopenia and neutropenia are so infrequent as to be possibly coincidental. Side effects are usually reversed by lowering the dose, and appear to be less frequent when the drug is started at low dosage and gradually increased.[38] The incremental method of beginning indomethacin administration is particularly helpful in averting severe headache, one of the most common causes of patient noncompliance.

In 1967 Jacobs reported the sudden deaths of two JRA patients who were receiving large doses of indomethacin, one of whom had received an exceptionally large dose (up to 9 mg/kg/day).[42] Septicemia was proven in one case and suspected in the other. At about the same time a case of fatal toxic hepatitis was reported in a 12-year-old boy who had been receiving indomethacin for JRA.[43] This patient was also treated with corticosteroids and aspirin, the latter a now proven hepatotoxin. Soon after these reports indomethacin was mandated by the FDA as contraindicated for use in children under 14 years of age. It should be noted, however, that the evidence implicating indomethacin in these deaths is circumstantial. The risk of death from infection may be generally increased in severe JRA,[44] and necropsy evidence of severe hepatitis is also frequent.[45]

Few investigations of the use of indomethacin in JRA have been carried out in this country but where these have been done the results were generally favorable. Indomethacin has clearly been shown to be superior to both acetaminaphen and placebo as an antipyretic agent in children.[46] Patterson used it in 57 children with JRA for periods up to 40 months in dosage ranging from 2 to 4 mg/kg/day, and occasionally as high as 6 mg/kg/day.[47] With indomethacin therapy elimination or reduction of concomitant corticosteroid therapy was possible in 21 of 26 children. These authors noted no evidence of drug-related hepatotoxicity, and no instances of severe infections, concluding that the drug was a safe and useful mode of therapy for JRA. Other authors have obtained similar results[48,49] which are generally in agreement with studies of adult RA patients which have shown the drug to be effective in controlling the disease, providing a steroid-sparing effect, and in enhancing the beneficial response in those patients receiving chrysotherapy.

The present authors feel that indomethacin is a useful antiinflammatory drug in some children with JRA. We have found it very effective in controlling the febrile manifestations of systemic JRA when maximal doses of salicylates fail to do so. In this situation indomethacin has sometimes been as effective as corticosteroids[50] and has enabled some patients with very toxic systemic JRA to be managed without steroid therapy. We have also used it in patients with severe polyarticular disease where gold therapy is not indicated or has not been effective. In no instance has hepatotoxicity or severe infection resulted. Although headaches and dyspepsia are not uncommon, by gradually titrating the dosage upward these have been kept to a minimum. Maintenance administration of 3 mg/kg/day, in three or four divided doses, with the total dose rarely exceeding 100 mg/day, is generally effective. Although studies have shown interaction between aspirin and indomethacin[51] with reduction of indomethacin plasma concentrations, there appears to be little clinical effect from this interaction and we commonly utilize both drugs in combination.

The potential side effects of indomethacin and its medicolegal status are such that it probably should be reserved for use in centers having extensive experience in the management of JRA.

CHRYSOTHERAPY

Aspirin and the rapid-acting antiinflammatory drugs discussed above are suitable standards against which other regimens can be measured. These medications are preferred for initial therapy because of ease of administration, tolerance by children, cost, and for most, safety. Although chrysotherapy requires parenteral administration and frequent clinic and laboratory visits the known efficacy and infrequency of severe adverse reactions makes gold therapy the logical choice when JRA is uncontrolled by aspirin or NSAIDs. In trials, reported almost 50 years ago gold compounds had been shown to inhibit the growth of tubercle bacilli in vitro, and were given to rheumatoid patients by Forestier because of histologic similarities between rheumatoid arthritis and tuberculosis.[52] During the next 30 years because of strongly suggested therapeutic efficacy interest in chrysotherapy remained high and many reports from this period document beneficial effects as well as a high potential for toxicity. It remained, however, for the Research Subcommittee of the Empire Rheumatism Council finally to publish the results of a controlled multicenter trial in 1960.[53]

Many early reports included a few children and subsequent series on JRA patients have now been published;[54-58] however, no controlled studies of chrysotherapy in JRA have been reported.

The heightened immunologic activity noted in JRA suggests that gold may act upon the immune system directly. Studies have shown that delayed and immediate hypersensitivity as determined by skin test reactions, and immunoglobulin production are not significantly altered by gold injections.[59] Further, although rheumatoid-factor titers fall in both adults[53] and children[60] during chrysotherapy, this is transient and does not correlate well with clinical improvement.

In contrast it can be demonstrated by skin window techniques and by introduction of peritoneal foreign bodies, that there is a dose-dependent inhibition of phagocytic activity by polymorphs and macrophages.[61,62] In the case of the macrophage, this is sustained in duration, and selective concentration of gold by synovial macrophages is suggested.[63] An additional observation from these studies is that the amount of interstitial fluid is decreased in gold-treated subjects, possibly representing a stabilization of capillary permeability.

Another potentially important mechanism is the effect of gold on enzymes capable of degrading the mucopolysaccharide matrix of cartilage. Prior reports of inhibition of acid phosphatase (and in some reports of beta-glucuronidase and cathepsin)[64] were considered suspect since the optimal pH for acid phosphatase is 3.0. The subsequent identification of a gold-sensitive neutral protease with demonstrable activity on cartilage made this hypothesis attractive.[65] Release of such enzymes is not impaired by gold but since gold can be found in the granular fraction of cells it is likely that intra- and extracellular enzyme inhibition occurs, presumably via the binding of sulfhydryl groups.

After intramuscular injection aqueous gold solutions are rapidly absorbed, reaching peak serum levels within eight hours; 95% of gold in serum can be localized to the albumin fraction. Gold levels in serum increase during the first four to six weeks of therapy and thereafter are relatively stable. The major route of excretion of gold is in the urine with fecal excretion in most studies accounting for smaller amounts.[66] Large amounts (up to 85%) of gold are retained and excreted very gradually over a period of months to years following discontinuation of long-term therapy.[67]

Our criteria for the initiation of gold therapy are: (1) severe systemic symptoms or joint disease which does not improve during six months of adequate aspirin or NSAID therapy, (2) progression of joint disease during six months of adequate aspirin therapy or NSAID therapy, and (3) corticosteroid dependence. These guidelines should be modified to individual needs. It may not be necessary to wait six months to begin injections in individuals in whom vigorous NSAID therapy is not effective. In some cases this may be apparent within two to three months. It is preferable to begin gold before resorting to daily corticosteroid therapy, although methylprednisolone "pulse therapy" may be useful (*vide infra*). In contrast to the rapid-acting antiinflammatory agents salutary effects do not appear before eight to 12 weeks of chrysotherapy.

Utilizing these criteria 125 children (14% of all JRA patients) with all modes of onset have been treated with gold at Children's Hospital of Los Angeles. Ninety-three percent of these patients had systemic or polyarticular onset of JRA. The remaining were children with pauciarticular-onset JRA which was unusually severe or had progressed to polyarticular involvement after the first six months of illness.

In this country gold has been most widely used as the aqueous compound; gold sodium thiomalate (Myochrysine). Although other preparations are available they are not in widespread clinical use and will not be considered in this discussion. Gold sodium thiomalate (GST) is 50% gold by weight and is available in 10, 25, 50, and 100 mg/ml dosage forms. Although these multiple concentrations are very useful in the pediatric clinic, extreme care must be used to avoid mistakes in selecting a preparation which would lead to an inadequate dose or more seriously, an overdose.

In our clinics chrysotherapy is initiated with progressively increasing test doses of 0.25 to 0.75 mg/kg/week for the first three weeks. If no toxicity is apparent weekly injections of 1 mg/kg/week are administered for 15 to 20 weeks depending on clinical response. In most centers the therapy course is 20 weekly injections followed by continued injections at two weeks and later, longer intervals. We have found that relapses occurring during therapy at two to four week intervals between injections have been poorly responsive to resumption of weekly chrysotherapy. For this reason we have continued weekly injections for longer periods than 20 weeks and proceeded with caution to two week intervals only when disease control is good. Only rarely are longer intervals utilized. Lacking controlled studies we have chosen complete absence of clinically active disease for one year as a suitable criterion for discontinuing therapy. This decision must be made on a more arbitrary basis, unless toxicity occurs, for patients without complete remission.

Additional laboratory studies are suggested prior to beginning and at intervals during gold therapy. These include: (1) quantitative immunoglobulins, (2) erythrocyte sedimentation rate, (3) reticulocyte count, and (4) liver enzymes.

The value of serum gold determinations remains controversial.[69,70] It is clear that the pharmacokinetics of gold are complicated, and thus determinations of serum gold levels are an indirect method of assessment of therapy. When serum drawn for gold levels seven days after the last injection are found to be low, particularly in the child with a poor or equivocal response to gold therapy after 12 weekly injections, small weekly dose increments may produce clinical improvement. Lorber's recommendation that serum levels be maintained at 300 to 350 μgm% is usually achieved at 1.25 mg/kg/week if a dose increase is required at all.[69] Doses in excess of 1.5 mg/kg/week are not recommended.

The considerable variations in study design, mechanics of administration, length of follow-up, and criteria for improvement make statistics describing outcome difficult to evaluate. Freyberg has summarized the experience from a number of major studies in adults.[67] The Empire Rheumatism Council Study established symptomatic and functional improvement in gold therapy compared to control subjects, and these observations have been confirmed.[53] The additional findings of fewer bone erosions and less joint space narrowing suggesting alteration of the natural history of RA has been more recently reported.[71] Although it is apparent that the majority of patients initially improve, often dramatically, it is also probable that toxic effects, limited improvement, nonresponse, or relapse eventually adversely affect the outcome in up to 60% of chrysotherapy patients.

The same difficulties that complicate outcome statistics from reports of RA are seen in reviews of the experience with chrysotherapy for JRA. The older literature indicates that overall prognosis may not be affected, but more recent publications indicate remission or marked improvement in approximately 40%, and less dramatic improvement in an additional 14 to 30% of patients.[54,57,58] Sairanen[56] reported improvement in sedimentation rate and articular index to be greater in gold-treated children than in controls; Hanson's[57] report indicates that functional class improved in 17 of 20 children in Class 2, and in seven of 16 children in Class 3.

There is great concern about the toxicity of gold therapy and the observation that up to 50% of patients receiving chrysotherapy will have adverse reactions validates this concern.[55,57] It must be recalled, however, that the majority of these reactions are mild or inconsequential and almost all are reversible without residua. Scrupulous adherence to the practice of careful history-taking, physical examinations, and review of laboratory data, will minimize the likelihood of serious adverse effects.

Prior to every injection an interval history and complete physical examination should be performed with emphasis on the skin for evidence of toxicity and joint status for serial evaluation. In addition all patients must have a weekly CBC and urinalysis evaluated prior to each injection. Our experience suggests that the following abnormalities are cause for alarm:

(1) total WBC below 5000/mm^3, or total neutrophil count (TNC) below 2000/mm^3,

(2) a 50% decrease in WBC or TNC compared with determinations from the previous week,

(3) proteinuria by dipstick of 2+ or greater,

(4) hematuria (particularly in combination with proteinuria),

(5) any unusual rash.

While the findings listed above demand recognition, choosing the appropriate course of action is sometimes difficult. Temporary cessation of injections when modest hematologic abnormalities appear is usually followed by a rapid recovery which should be documented by repeat blood counts two or three times weekly. Gold injections may then be resumed starting with a small test dose and progressing in increments as is done when initiating therapy.

Some clinicians have found that continuation of gold therapy with mild to moderate dermatitis is possible.[69] Seven to 33% of reactions in children involve the skin and mucosal surfaces (usually the mouth). Cheilosis and mucosal lesions may occur but have not, in our experience, been accompanied by complaints of metallic taste as is often described in adult patients. Clinically, the cutaneous eruptions are most often pruritic erythematous papules or macules, but these may be described as lichen planus or pityriasis rosea. Generalized exfoliative dermatitis occurs but is rare in our experience. Erythema nodosum and urticarial drug eruptions are also described. Histologically, inflammatory perivascular infiltrates of lymphocytes, macrophages, plasma cells, and sometimes neutrophils are often prominent, or edema and infiltration with eosinophils may be seen.[72] Serum IgE elevations indicate a type I hypersensitivity reaction.[73] Recovery is the rule although this may require months to years to be complete. Gold injections have been resumed at lower doses or at greater intervals between injections without recurrence.

There is a broad spectrum of hematologic manifestations of gold toxicity ranging from apparently benign eosinophilia to catastrophic and fatal aplastic anemias; fortunately the latter are very rare. The most frequently seen complication is that of mild to moderate depression of granulocytes which responds rapidly to discontinuance of gold within a period of weeks. Thrombocytopenia appears more commonly in adults than children and may be more persistent in duration. Severe neutropenia occurs more frequently in children than in adults but if infections are identified and treated early the complication is self-limited.[76] The mechanism of these reactions is uncertain but direct marrow depression seems likely in neutropenia and aplastic anemia.[74] Antibody mediation of thrombocytopenia has been suggested but remains undocumented.[75] If chrysotherapy is resumed following recovery from mild hematologic abnormalities, progressively increasing test doses should be used. The value of treating gold toxicity with dimercaprol is uncertain, and most cases do not require chelation therapy, although patients with persistent thrombocytopenia may be exceptions.[77]

Conversely, even in the absence of overt toxicity the potential marrow suppression[74] and inhibition of phagocytic function[61,62] is a theoretic handicap to children with intercurrent infections and temporary discontinuation of injections is suggested in these patients.

Among children renal toxicity represents 5% to more than 20% of the total toxic reactions reported during gold therapy. It is likely that causes of hematuria and proteinuria other than gold therapy have falsely elevated these figures. However, it is advisable to discontinue therapy in the presence of these signs if they cannot be accounted for by menses or other *known* causes. Nephritis, particularly in children with systemic-onset JRA, is one such cause of hematuria, and may be aggravated by aspirin therapy.[68] Serial urinalyses prior to beginning chrysotherapy will establish a baseline. Larger amounts of hematuria suggest that the discontinuance of gold injections is necessary, particularly when proteinuria is also present. However, massive proteinuria and the nephrotic syndrome have occurred in association with a membranous glomerulonephritis; prolonged proteinuria has been correlated with basement membrane thickening.[78] These findings suggest that GST should always be discontinued upon discovery of proteinuria. With this approach no serious renal sequelae have been observed in our gold-treated patients, and therapy has been resumed in several instances without return of urinary sediment changes.

The status of gold as a hepatotoxin is uncertain. Since toxic hepatitis may occur concomitant with systemic-onset JRA or secondary to a number of drugs used in the treatment of JRA it is difficult to determine the incidence of liver toxicity due to gold alone. Elevations of the transaminases usually respond with normalization to discontinuing the more common offending drugs such as aspirin. Marked or persistent elevation of liver enzyme levels should be observed with serial determinations and gold injections should be temporarily withheld.

Vasomotor (nitritoid) reactions characterized by generalized erythema, warmth, giddiness, blurred vision, and vertigo occur infrequently during the early weeks of therapy. The remaining toxic reactions such as enterocolitis, pneumonitis, keratitis, and corneal chrysiasis are very uncommon, and the causative role of gold is uncertain for some.

The foregoing discussion emphasizes the role of chrysotherapy in the treatment of JRA. Relative to aspirin and NSAIDs gold therapy is more expensive and time-consuming for both patient and physician. Further, children are predictably disturbed by injections, and potential morbidity and rarely, mortality can occur secondary to toxic reactions. As noted above, however, adverse reactions are almost always reversible and their occurrence can be minimized by careful physician scrutiny. The rewards are a high frequency of longlasting improvement or in some cases, remission. For patients already receiving oral corticosteroids an improvement with gold therapy may be the key to substantially lower doses or discontinuance of corticosteroids.

ANTIMALARIALS

Following reports by Page[79] and Freedman[80] that the antimalarial drugs of the 4-aminoquinoline class were able to suppress rheumatoid synovitis, their use became widespread in the treatment of rheumatoid arthritis. Hydroxychloroquine sulfate (Plaquenil) is the quinoline derivative now most frequently used since it has a lower incidence of side effects and is apparently equal in efficacy to chloroquine phosphate (Aralen).[38] Hydroxychloroquine is rapidly and completely absorbed following oral administration. Plasma concentration increases rapidly during the first week of therapy, and then more slowly so that final equilibrium is attained after four to six weeks. Although plasma levels remain low, concentration of drug in the tissues is very high, with levels in the liver, spleen, kidney, and lung being 400 to 700 times that of plasma.[38] Excretion is slow, and detectable amounts of chloroquine have been found in urine, red cells, and plasma of patients with retinopathy as long as five years after the last ingestion of the drug.[81]

The mechanism of action of the antimalarial drugs is still not clearly understood. Unlike other more rapidly acting antiinflammatory agents, they do not have analgesic or antipyretic effects.[82] The antiinflammatory effects of antimalarials may be related to their known concentration in lysosomes, perhaps resulting in stabilization of lysosomal membranes, and in their ability directly to inhibit both the chemotactic and phagocytic functions of polymorphonuclear leukocytes.[83,84]

The most frequent side effects of the antimalarial drugs are ocular complications, bleaching and loss of hair, anorexia, abdominal discomfort, and neuromuscular weakness.[38] Major side effects in normal clinical use, however, have been ocular manifestations. Keratopathy is most common but relatively mild and reversible when the drug is stopped. Of more concern has been a retinopathy beginning with macular edema and occasionally continuing to progress even after treatment has been discontinued. This retinopathy is generally dose-related, with a threshold dose for hydroxychloroquine being over 7.5 mg/kg/day.[85] In our experience this complication is very rare and can be avoided with a combination of attention to dosage and close monitoring by an ophthalmologist.

Deaths have occurred as a result of ingestion of a single large dose of chloroquine.[82] Children seem to be unusually sensitive to the lethal effect of large doses and fatalities have occurred with ingestion of as little as one gram. Death occurs as a result of cardiorespiratory arrest; prompt treatment using mechanical ventilation and cardiac monitoring may be life-saving.[86]

Several double-blind studies in adults with RA show clear but moderate improvement in disease activity.[87] The drug appears to be cumulative in action, requiring several weeks to exert its beneficial effect and several months before maximal effects are obtained. There are no controlled studies of antimalarial therapy in JRA. Brewer[50] believes that chloroquine should not be used in children because of its potential ocular side effects, but Ansell[88] uses antimalarials for periods up to two years in children when gold cannot be given. Laaksonen et al. studied 119 children with JRA and found hydroxychloroquine to be safe in dosages up to 7 mg/kg/day.[89]

The present authors have found hydroxychloroquine to be a useful medication for selected JRA patients. These have been children with active progressive disease in spite of adequate therapy with the faster-acting antiinflammatory drugs, where for whatever reasons, gold therapy can not be employed, and where the child is not sufficiently ill to warrant the use of an experimental drug such as D-penicillamine. In such instances we have used doses of 3 to 5 mg/kg/day, and have always added hydroxychloroquine to the therapeutic regimen rather than stopping other medications. Any subsequent disease exacerbations have generally been handled by increasing or changing the faster-acting drugs rather than hydroxychloroquine. Baseline ophthalmologic examinations are obtained at the institution of therapy and every three to four months thereafter. Maintaining the above doses and periodic eye examinations no instances of retinopathy have resulted in our clinic.

Since hydroxychloroquine appears to produce stabilization of lysosomal membranes and gold therapy may inhibit the reaction of the lysosomal enzymes, there may be a rationale for the use of the two drugs in combination. Obviously frequent clinical and laboratory observations of children treated in this fashion will be essential to observe for possible cumulative toxicities of concomitant therapy. A prospective study of hydroxychloroquine as an adjunctive medication for the treatment of JRA is clearly needed.

PENICILLAMINE

Penicillamine first received attention for the treatment of rheumatoid disease following a 1964 report by Jaffe.[90] The most prominent previous uses of penicillamine had been for the therapy of Wilson's disease, cystinuria, and certain heavy metal intoxications. Originally, the D-L-penicillamine isomer was employed until it became evident that at least some of the severe toxicities, such as nephrotic syndrome, optic neuritis, and bone marrow suppression, could be reduced by using only the D-penicillamine isomer (B, B-dimethylcysteine).

Several large well controlled studies of the efficacy of penicillamine in adult rheumatoid arthritis have been performed,[91-93] and it now has limited application in the general practice of rheumatology. Zuckner and coworkers[92] treated 15 patients and observed all to have a fall in titer of rheumatoid factor (RF), most to have a decrease in sedimentation rate, and several to have an improvement in ARA functional class.[92] The English multicentre trial group studied 30 patients with advanced rheumatoid disease in a 12-month double-blind trial and showed statistically significant improvement in pain, morning gel, articular index, and functional assessment. Sera from these latter patients were independently studied by Bluestone and Goldberg who demonstrated a significant fall in IgG and IgM levels, but not IgA, and a significant fall in latex agglutination RF titers, but not those done by sheep cell agglutination.

The mechanisms by which penicillamine affects immunologic and clinical change are not known. The drug is known in vitro to disrupt interchain disulphide bonds of macroglobulins, although this may not occur in vivo. Many consider penicillamine to be immunosuppressive, but its variety of actions elucidated in the laboratory do not fully document why it is clinically effective.

The potential for significant toxicity remains a major concern for most investigators and practitioners who employ penicillamine therapy. Rash, thrombocytopenia, and proteinuria are prominent concerns, but loss of taste, anorexia, nausea, and vomiting also occasionally occur.[92,93] Optic neuritis appears to occur less frequently than previously, but induction of an SLE-like syndrome has been reported. Immune complex induction of nephritis and perhaps other toxic manifestations, and idiosyncratic hypersensitivity both may occur in addition to immunosuppressive manifestations. In some situations, penicillamine may be withdrawn and restarted at lower doses without toxicity reoccurrence, or short courses of corticosteroids may be used with or without stopping the penicillamine. The suggestion of Jaffe to begin therapy in steplike increments appears helpful, but a major difficulty is lack of certainty regarding the minimum effective dose.[94]

Penicillamine therapy has also been employed in essential cryoglobulinemia, autoimmune hemolytic anemia, and most particularly, in scleroderma,[95] because of evidence suggesting penicillamine's ability to increase the solubility of dermal collagen, and decrease intramolecular cross-linking.[96]

This drug has only recently been used for JRA and must be considered investigational. The most extensive experience is that of Ansell and coworkers whose findings and anecdotal observations from others experienced with JRA suggest that penicillamine is roughly comparable to gold in efficacy, but monitoring for toxicities must be done carefully.[97] At the Children's Hospital of Los Angeles an investigational penicillamine protocol has enrolled 10 children with JRA who were resistant to all more conventional forms of therapy. The benefit/risk ratio appears acceptable but it is too early for the presentation of meaningful data about efficacy. It can be strongly urged that the present use of penicillamine in children with JRA should be restricted to academic centers where a detailed study protocol is in force, and where reasonable numbers of patients can be systematically studied.

CORTICOSTEROIDS

Great excitement and speculation that a cure was at hand greeted the introduction of corticosteroids to the treatment of rheumatoid arthritis in 1949.[98] Initially there was great enthusiasm for their use in both adult RA and JRA.[99] But as is so often the case with new methods of treatment, further research and clinical experience brought the realization that corticosteroids, although the most potent of antiinflammatory drugs, did not provide a cure for the disease and in many instances acted to the patient's disadvantage. In 1956 Ansell[100] reported no difference between salicylate therapy and early steroid therapy in JRA while others have reported upon the many side effects of even low dose long-term steroid therapy in childhood.[101]

Although the corticosteroids are undoubtedly the most potent antiinflammatory agents known their many undesirable side effects are such that their use should be reserved only for specific indications in the treatment of JRA. Since much has been written about these side effects we will not detail them except to emphasize our major concern about their retardant effect upon normal growth.[102] Long-term, daily prednisone in dosage exceeding 5 mg/M²/day has been clearly shown to produce growth retardation.[103] Furthermore corticosteroid therapy in JRA does not prevent progression of joint narrowing, deformity, and destruction and there is even evidence that steroid therapy may lead to more severe joint damage due to possible interference with cartilage nutrition and avascular necrosis.[104] Nonetheless, steroid therapy does provide impressive short term benefits often bringing prompt relief of joint pain and swelling, defervescence of fever, and subjective improvement.

It is the authors' strong belief that corticosteroids should never be employed as the first treatment of JRA. Unfortunately it is not uncommon for the child with mild or moderate JRA to be referred to us after having been placed on a corticosteroid regimen which was either clinically not indicated or where an adequate trial of nonsteroidal drugs had not been administered. These children frequently manifested side effects of therapy which were out of proportion to the severity of their JRA. Our practice in such cases is to taper and discontinue the steroids but this may be very difficult due to dependence which frequently leads to increased disease manifestations when therapy is withdrawn. Successful steroid discontinuation often requires many months of extremely slow dose tapering, and often concomitant therapy with alternative drugs. It may be difficult to convince parents that the increased discomfort which their child may undergo during this period is a necessary price to pay. Thus the family must be well-educated about the risks of ongoing corticosteroid therapy, since any lack of understanding may end in their refusal to cooperate with steroid tapering and a resultant cushingoid permanently dwarfed child.

In addition to the danger of disease exacerbation during steroid reduction it must be remembered that adrenal insufficiency may develop during periods of intense stress, including administration of anesthesia for even relatively minor surgical procedures.[105] This period of relative adrenal insufficiency may persist for many months following total discontinuation of steroids, and children subject to stress should therefore be given appropriate steroid booster doses. It is our practice to administer "steroid preps" prior to, during, and following anesthesia, in any patient who has been on steroid therapy with a one and one-half year period previously.

In the authors' opinion corticosteroid therapy for JRA should be administered only under certain specific conditions. These include the following:

(1) Life-threatening disease. Most JRA fatalities have occurred as a result of complications such as severe infection, hepatic failure and, very rarely in North America, amyloidosis.[44,106] However myocarditis does occur in about 10% of patients with systemic JRA.[107] Since it has the potential to produce congestive failure, arrythmias, or cardiac arrest, myocarditis must be considered potentially life-threatening. Pericarditis, on the other hand, is rarely life-threatening and in most cases can be treated with other antiinflammatory drugs.[107] Severe pericarditis, however, warrants steroid therapy since it may result in pericardial tamponade. In such instances, high dosages (prednisolone 60 to 70 mg/M^2/day in divided doses) may be valuable.

(2) Iridocyclitis. Early and relatively mild eye disease is appropriately treated with topical steroids and dilating agents. Severe progressive iridocyclitis may, however, result in permanent visual deficit or blindness and a course of systemic corticosteroid therapy may be effective in such children.[50] Of particular concern in such patients, however, is the risk that posterior subcapsular cataracts, a known side effect of corticosteroid therapy, may be even more severe than those which may result from topical steroid therapy alone.[108]

(3) Children with severe, debilitating disease whose activities are profoundly limited and who have not responded to other antiinflammatory drugs. There do seem to be some children to whom a small dosage of corticosteroid (less than 10 mg prednisolone/day) may be the difference between being virtually bedridden, or being up and about and able to attend school. The problem is that it may be very difficult to determine those children in whom such small dosage will achieve the goal of significant functional improvement. In many cases following initial improvement, disease manifestations subsequently increase and higher doses of steroids are required. Before long these children are having significant side effects and it becomes very difficult to taper their steroids without disease flare-up. Here a relatively short-term course of corticosteroid therapy may be effective in maintaining function during the time that it takes for a slow-acting antiinflammatory

drug, such as gold, to become effective. The institution of steroids for this third group should be done only after consultation with a physician experienced in pediatric rheumatology. It is imperative that the plan of treatment for any child placed on systemic steroid therapy be eventually to withdraw such treatment.

Several methods of obtaining the beneficial effects of corticosteroids, while minimizing adverse effects have been tried. It is known that there is less adrenal suppression and fewer side effects with alternate-day steroid therapy.[109,110] This has been used in severe JRA and in some instances has been effective.[111] However, there is a tendency for the disease to exacerbate on the "off" day with uncontrollable fever spikes towards the end of the 48-hour period between steroid doses particularly troublesome in the systemic patient. It may be possible to control these by using higher doses of aspirin or indomethacin on the off day. In other cases, because of the severity of the disease alternate-day therapy is not practical. Another situation where alternate-day therapy may be useful, however, is during steroid reduction. Divided daily doses may first be changed to a single daily dose, then converted to alternate-day therapy, and finally slowly reduced in dosage.

ACTH therapy has been felt by some to produce fewer side effects, and in particular less growth retardation than the corticosteroids.[112] We have not noted any significant difference in either efficacy or adverse effects between corticosteroids and ACTH therapy.

A third, recent technique of steroid utilization has been termed "pulse therapy." This consists of giving massive doses of a potent glucocorticoid, usually methylprednisolone, intravenously at 30 mg/kg, on three consecutive days, no more frequently than once a month. We have treated approximately 15 JRA patients and a number of systemic lupus patients in this manner and in no instance have clinical signs of adrenal suppression or the expected side effects of long-term steroid therapy resulted. In one case there was a transient period of hypotension which was asymptomatic and resolved spontaneously after a few minutes. There have been no instances of hypertension or apparent fluid retention, all patients showing a marked reduction in the signs and symptoms of their disease as expected, immediately following therapy. One child with previously uncontrollable systemic JRA has gone into a long-term remission which has now lasted many months. The other children had much more transient amelioration of their disease, and in some cases relief of symptoms lasted only several days. For this reason we now use pulse therapy less frequently. It may, however, be a useful means of buying time without producing steroid side effects in the child with severe disease who is being started on gold therapy.

Although systemic steroid therapy has a very limited role in the treatment of JRA, local steroid therapy is often very useful. Steroid eye drops along with dilating agents are effective in controlling many cases of iridocyclitis, particularly when treatment is begun early.[113] Intraarticular steroid injection can also be very useful particularly when only one or a small number of joints are inflamed and producing symptoms. In some instances where many joints are involved one or two may be particularly troublesome, and intraarticular steroids may make the child much more functional. One joint which we are reluctant to inject, however, is the hip joint since the femoral head is particularly susceptible to avascular necrosis.

The least soluble and longest-acting preparation for injection appears to be triamcinalone hexacetonide. Single injections have often resulted in complete resolution of the clinical signs of inflammation for many months but this preparation may frequently, by infiltration, produce atrophy and scarring of the subcutaneous tissues. For this reason we rarely use it for injecting superficial or more highly visible joints such as fingers, wrists, or ankles. Repeated or too frequent use of the long-acting preparations has also been reported to lead to a crystal-induced synovitis. Although its effects are not as long lasting, for smaller or more visible joints we frequently use triamcinalone acetonide which produces a relatively prolonged reduction in joint inflammation.

Careful aseptic technique must be used whenever a joint is being injected. Except when a joint effusion is very large we generally do not aspirate fluid prior to injecting steroids. If, however, there is the slightest suspicion of joint sepsis, appropriate synovial fluid studies should be performed and steroid injection deferred until infection is eliminated as a diagnostic possibility. It should be remembered that a rheumatoid joint may be even more susceptible to infection than a normal joint, therefore one should not automatically conclude that worsening inflammation of a JRA joint is always due to rheumatoid disease exacerbation.

IMMUNOSUPPRESSIVE THERAPY

Immunosuppressive therapy in rheumatoid disease is an experimental form of treatment aimed at modifying the immune system, derangement of which may be important in the pathogenesis of the disease. These methods attempt to alter the pathologic chain of events at an earlier stage in pathogenesis than the previously discussed antiinflammatory agents. Immunosuppresive therapy, as with all other drug types, is nonspecific since it is not directed at the cause of the disease, and because it may inhibit useful as well as harmful immune and inflammatory responses.

The major immunosuppressive drugs used for RA have been the alkylating agents (cyclophosphamide and chlorambucil, both nitrogen mustards), and the antimetabolite, azathioprine (a purine analog). Methotrexate, a folic acid inhibitor, has been more often used in the treatment of psoriatic arthritis and dermatomyositis,[114,115] and only infrequently for RA.

Cyclophosphamide and chlorambucil reacting directly with nucleoprotein and DNA, cause denaturation and disrupted protein synthesis, and thus interfere with the normal mitosis and cell division of all rapidly proliferating tissues. Their immunosuppressive effects are considered to be due to the particular sensitivity of lymphocytes to their destructive action.[116]

Azathioprine is a derivative of 6-mercaptopurine (6-MP) and reacts with sulfhydryl groups to cause the slow liberation of free 6-MP which displays superior immunosuppressive activity in comparison with the parent compound.[117] The purine analogues are incorporated into nucleic acids and inhibit intermediate nucleotide metabolism, leading to cell death. Based upon animal studies and its effect of preventing organ graft rejection in humans, it has been suggested that azathoprine has a predominant effect on the T-lymphocyte.[118]

Only a small number of controlled studies of immunosuppressive therapy for RA have been reported; as yet there have been no controlled trials in JRA. In a study of 48 patients with severe RA, 20 received a high dose of cyclophosphamide (up to 150 mg daily), and 28 a low dose (up to 15 mg daily) for 32 weeks.[119] A significant reduction in disease activity resulted in the high dose group as compared to the low dose group. Of particular interest was the finding that bone destruction, observed by serial radiographs, progressed in approximately one-half of the low dose group, but only one or two high dose patients showed progression of bone lesions. The authors concluded that cyclophosphamide produced a substantial improvement in RA but its hazards are such as to warrant its use only where more standard forms of therapy have failed.

Chlorambucil has undergone extensive clinical trials in France with good or excellent results in 50 to 80% of cases.[120] It has also been effective in some cases of intractable idiopathic uveitis.[121] Chlorambucil is considered to be the slowest-acting and least toxic of the nitrogen mustards; however, fatalities due to irreversible aplastic anemia have been reported.[122] The authors propose the following guidelines for its use: (1) patients with previous hematologic depression with any drug should have a bone marrow biopsy prior to chlorambucil therapy to insure adequate marrow reserves; (2) in patients developing leukopenia on chlorambucil, resumption of therapy should be withheld until leukocyte counts return to normal; (3) in patients with slow or inadequate resolution of drug-induced leukopenia, bone marrow biopsy should be performed before resuming chlorambucil.

Both cyclophosphamide and chlorambucil share the hazards of bone marrow depression, increased risk of infection, alopecia, and infertility due to azoospermia and ovarian failure.[123,124] In addition all of the immunosuppressive drugs may increase the risks of later developing neoplasia. Generally, however, chlorambucil appears to be less toxic than cyclophosphamide and has the added advantage of not causing the hemorrhagic cystitis which is a frequent severe, early or late complication of cyclophosphamide therapy.

Azathioprine has been investigated in 17 adults with severe RA using a double-blind crossover study method during two 16 week periods.[125] Subsequently this study was extended in 12 of the original 17 patients as an open trial for a mean period of 40 months.[126] The authors found a significant improvement in the azathioprine group during the double-blind phase of the study which was maintained during the long term portion. Although adverse side effects were minor an increased incidence of chromosomal abnormalities was detected. Azathioprine was also used in the treatment of 13 children (age two to 13 years) with severe active JRA.[127] It was felt to be effective, occasionally strikingly so, in the majority of patients; no control group was studied for comparison.

Azathioprine hepatotoxicity has been a relatively frequent side effect but is usually reversible when treatment is stopped. Leukopenia has been less common than with the alkylating agents; an increased incidence of neoplasia is reported in patients who received azathioprine with renal allografts.[128]

The authors have utilized cyclophosphamide and chlorambucil in the treatment of selected children with JRA. Treatment criteria have included severe active disease which has been refractory to standard antiinflammatory agents as well as, in some instances, to d-penicillamine. Patients must have had radiologic evidence of progressive joint destruction for more than one year. Most of these children were also having severe toxicity from corticosteroids. Cyclophosphamide (approximately 2 mg/kg/day), and chlorambucil (0.1 to 0.2 mg/kg/day), both produced improvement and, in some cases, clinical remission of disease when therapy could be maintained for periods of three months or more. Leukopenia forced dose reduction or cessation in some instances. A major problem with cyclophosphamide was hemorrhagic cystitis, including persistence in some children for long periods following therapy. One girl still has cystitis, with characteristic bladder findings on cystoscopy five years after the cessation of therapy. Another girl with systemic lupus erythematosus treated with cyclophosphamide required instillation of formalin into her bladder to control life-threatening hemorrhage.

The major side effects produced by chlorambucil in our patients have been thrombocytopenia and leukopenia; bone marrow recovery has occurred in all instances following cessation of therapy. As little as 2 mg of chlorambucil per day appears to be providing excellent control of disease in some patients, and all who have been able to tolerate therapy have shown improvement.

The potentially life-threatening hazards of therapy with these cytotoxic agents must be carefully weighed in the selection of suitable candidates for their use. Consideration must be given not only to the more immediate side effects such as bone marrow depression, but also to the potential late effects such as infertility, possible genetic aberrations in the patients' offspring, and risk of malignancy eventually developing. In a child with many years of life ahead and where risk of mortality from disease is not great, the decision to embark on immunosuppressive therapy is a particularly difficult one.

CONCLUSION

The drug therapy of JRA is currently directed towards the amelioration of signs and symptoms of the disease, primarily by nonspecific suppression of the inflammatory response, rather than towards etiologic mechanisms. This reality, forced by our lack of knowledge of etiology, provides effective relief in many cases but must be considered an inadequate alternative. New therapeutic techniques currently under investigation such as levamisole and transfer factor may provide more specific regulation of dysfunctional components of the immune system, but they too lack precision because of our fundamental lack of understanding of causative factors. Clearly more rational therapy for JRA must await further developments in clinical and basic research to provide more specific answers about genetic, environmental, or infectious aspects of pathogenesis.

REFERENCES

1. Gross, M., and Greenberg, L.A. *The Salicylates—A Critical Bibliographic Review*. New Haven, Connecticut: Hillhouse Press, 1948.
2. Fremont-Smith, K. Metabolism, pharmacology, and toxicology of salicylates. Edited by R.W. Lamont-Havers and B.M. Wagner. In *Proceedings*

of the Conference on Effects of Chronic Salicylate Administration. U.S. Department of Health, Education, and Welfare, Bethesda, Md.: 1966, pp. 1–5.

3. Leonards, J.R. Metabolism, pharmacology, and toxicology of salicylates. Edited by R.W. Lamont-Havers and B.M. Wagner. In Proceedings of the Conference on Effects of Chronic Salicylate Administration. U.S. Department of Health, Education, and Welfare, Bethesda, Md.: 1966, pp. 5–14.

4. Woodbury, D.M. Analgesic-antipyretics, antiinflammatory agents, and inhibitors of uric acid synthesis. Edited by L.S. Goodman and A.G. Gilman. In The Pharmacological Basis of Therapeutics. 4th ed. New York: MacMillan Company, 1970, pp. 314–29.

5. Pachman, L., Esterle, N.B., and Peterson, R.D.A. The effect of salicylate on the metabolism of normal and stimulated human lymphocytes in vitro. J Clin Invest. 50:226–30, 1971.

6. Duncan, M.W., Person, D.A., Rich, R.R., and Sharp, J.T. Aspirin and delayed type hypersensitivity. Arthritis Rheum. 20:1174–8, 1977.

7. Vane, J.R. Inhibition of prostaglandin synthesis as a mechanism of action for aspirin-like drugs. Nature (New Biology). 231:232–5, 1971.

8. Flower, R.M. Drugs which inhibit prostaglandin-biosynthesis. Pharmacol Rev. 26:33–67, 1974.

9. Levy, G. Biopharmaceutical aspects of the gastrointestinal absorption of salicylates. Edited by A. St. J. Dixon, et al. In Salicylates, an International Symposium. Boston: Little, Brown, and Co. 1963, pp. 10–16.

10. Klinenberg, J.R., and Miller, F. Effect of corticosteroids on blood salicylate concentration. JAMA. 194:131–4, 1965.

11. Bernstein, B.H., Singsen, B.H., Koster, K.K., and Hanson, V. Aspirin induced hepatotoxicity and its effect on juvenile rheumatoid arthritis. Am J Dis Child. 131:659–63, 1977.

12. Miller, J.J., III, and Weissmann, D.B. Correlation between transaminase concentrations and serum salicylate concentrations in juvenile rheumatoid arthritis. Arthritis Rheum. 19:115–18, 1976.

13. Gordon, J.L., and MacIntyre, D.E. Inhibition of human platelet aggregation by aspirin in vitro and in vivo. Br J Pharmacol. 52:451, 1974.

14. Levinson, J.E., Baum, J., Brewer, E. Jr. et al. Comparison of tolmetin sodium and aspirin in the treatment of juvenile rheumatoid arthritis. J Pediatr. 90:799–804, 1977.

15. Plostnieks, J., Cressman, W.A., Lemanowicz, E.F. et al. Human metabolism of tolmetin. Edited by J. Ward. In Tolmetin, a New Nonsteroidal Antiinflammatory Agent. Excerpta Medica, International Congress Series 372. New York: American Elsevier, 1975, pp. 23–33.

16. Ferreira, S.H., and Vane, J.R. New aspects of mode of action of nonsteroid antiinflammatory drugs. Ann Rev Pharmacol. 14:57–73, 1974.

17. Johnson, P.C., Lindsky, M., and Amodio, P., Jr. Evaluation of the endocrine system response to tolmetin in patients with acute rheumatoid arthritis. Edited by J. Ward. In Tolmetin, a New Nonsteroidal Antiinflammatory Agent. Excerpta Medica, International Congress Series 372. New York: American Elsevier, 1975, pp. 184–99.

18. Johnson, H.H., Herzog, J.P., and Lauler, D.P. Effect of prostaglandin E_1 on renal hemodynamics, sodium and water excretion. Am J Physiol. 213:939–46, 1967.

19. Mielke, C.H., Jr., Heiden, D., and Amodio, P., Jr. Tolmetin: hematological effects in normal subjects. Edited by J. Ward. In Tolmetin, a

New Nonsteroidal Antiinflammatory Agent. Excerpta Medica, International Congress Series 372. New York: American Elsevier, 1975, pp. 200–8.

20. Johnson, P.C. Gastrointestinal blood loss from antiinflammatory agents. Edited by J. Ward. In *Tolmetin, a New Nonsteroidal Antiinflammatory Agent.* Excerpta Medica, International Congress Series 372, New York: American Elsevier, 1975, pp. 168–73.

21. Bernhard, G.C., Poiley, J., and Tarpley, E.L. A double-blind cooperative trial of tolmetin plus gold in the treatment of rheumatoid arthritis. Edited by J. Ward. In *Tolmetin, a New Nonsteroidal Antiinflammatory Agent.* Excerpta Medica, International Congress Series 372. New York: American Elsevier, 1975, pp. 122–32.

22. Roth, S.H., Englund, D.W., Harris, B.K., and Ross, H.A. Tolmetin with acetominophen in the treatment of rheumatoid arthritis. Edited by J. Ward. In *Tolmetin, a New Nonsteroidal Antiinflammatory Agent.* Excerpta Medica, International Congress Series 372. New York: American Elsevier, 1975, pp. 113–21.

23. Gruber, C.M., Jr. Clinical pharmacology of fenoprofen: a review. *J Rheumatol.* 3 (suppl 2):8–17, 1976.

24. Zuckner, J., and Auclair, J.J. Fenoprofen calcium therapy in rheumatoid arthritis. *J Rheumatol.* 3 (suppl 2):18–25, 1976.

25. Huskisson, E.C. Long term use of fenoprofen in rheumatoid arthritis: the therapeutic ratio. *Curr Med Res Opin.* 2:545–50, 1974.

26. Gum, O.B. Fenoprofen in rheumatoid arthritis: a controlled crossover multicenter study. *J Rheumatol.* 3 (suppl 2):26–31, 1976.

27. Royer, G.L., Moxley, T.E., Hearron, M.S. et al. A long term double-blind clinical trial of ibuprofen and indomethacin in rheumatoid arthritis. *J Int Med Res.* 3:158–71, 1975.

28. Davies, E.F., and Avery, G.S. Ibuprofen: a review of pharmacological properties and therapeutic efficacy in rheumatic disorders. *Drugs.* 2:416–46, 1971.

29. Runkel, R., Chaplin, M., Boost, G. et al. Absorption, distribution, metabolism, and excretion of naproxen in various laboratory animals and human subjects. *J Pharm Sci.* 61:703–8, 1972.

30. Segre, E., Sevelius, H., Chaplin, M. et al. Interaction of naproxen and aspirin in the rat and in man. *Scand J Rheumatol.* (suppl 2):37–42, 1973.

31. Helby-Peterson, P., Ilfelt, H., and Rossel, I. A double-blind cross-over comparison of naproxen and placebo in rheumatoid arthritis. *Scand J Rheumatol.* (suppl 2):145–9, 1973.

32. Hill, H.F.H., Hill, A.G.S., Mowat, A.G. et al. Naproxen. A new nonhormonal antiinflammatory agent. *Ann Rheum Dis.* 33:12–19, 1974.

33. Nadel, J., Bruno, J., Varady, J., and Segre, E.J. Effect of naproxen and of aspirin on bleeding time and platelet time and platelet aggregation. *J Clin Pharmacol.* 14:176–82, 1974.

34. Norcross, B.M. Treatment of connective tissue disease with a new nonsteroidal compound (indomethacin), abstracted. *Arthritis Rheum.* 6:290, 1963.

35. Mainland, D. The Cooperating Clinics Committee of the American Rheumatism Association. A three month trial of indomethacin in rheumatoid arthritis, with special reference to analysis and inference. *Clin Pharmacol Ther.* 8:11–37, 1967.

36. Smyth, C.J. Indomethacin in rheumatoid arthritis. A comparative objective evaluation with adrenocorticosteroids. *Arthritis Rheum.* 8:921–42, 1965.

37. Kunze, M., Stein, G., Kunze, E., and Traeger, A. The pharmacokinetics of indomethacin in relation to age, in patients with occlusion of bile ducts, with reduced renal function, and with signs of intolerance. *Deut Gesundheitsw.* 29:351–3, 1974.

38. Lockie, L.M. Phenylbutazone, indomethacin and chloroquine in therapy of rheumatoid arthritis. Edited by J.L. Hollander. In *Arthritis and Allied Conditions*. 8th ed. Philadelphia: Lea and Febiger, 1972, pp. 483–94.

39. Vane, J.R. Prostaglandins and the aspirin-like drugs. *Hosp Prac.* 7:61–71, 1972.

40. O'Brien, W.M. Indomethacin: a survey of clinical trials. *Clin Pharmacol Ther.* 9:94–107, 1968.

41. Burns, C.A. Indomethacin, reduced retinal sensitivity and corneal deposits. *Am J Ophthalmol.* 66:825–35, 1968.

42. Jacobs, J.C. Sudden death in arthritic children receiving large doses of indomethacin. *JAMA.* 199:182–4, 1967.

43. Kelsey, W.M., and Scharyj, M. Fatal hepatitis probably due to indomethacin. *JAMA.* 199:154–5, 1967.

44. Bernstein, B. Death in juvenile rheumatoid arthritis. *Arthritis Rheum.* 20 (suppl):256–7, 1977.

45. Boone, J.E. Hepatic disease and mortality in juvenile rheumatoid arthritis. *Arthritis Rheum.* 20 (suppl):257–8, 1977.

46. Brewer, E.J., Jr. A comparative evaluation of indomethacin, acetaminophen, and placebo as antipyretic agents in children. *Arthritis Rheum.* 11:645–51, 1968.

47. Patterson, J.H., Tyston, W.R., and Gay, B.B. Indomethacin in the treatment of juvenile rheumatoid arthritis. In *Eighth International Congress of Pediatrics*. F. Feilhaur, Neunkirechen: Austria, 1971, pp. 175–82.

48. Roth, S.H., and Englund, D.W. Indomethacin in the treatment of juvenile rheumatoid arthritis. *Arthritis Rheum.* 10:307–8, 1967.

49. Sänger, L., Stoeber, E., and Kölle, G. Long term therapy with indomethacin in juvenile rheumatoid arthritis and Still's disease. *Arzneimittelforsch.* 17:1414–20, 1967.

50. Brewer, E.J., Jr. Drug therapy. Edited by E.J. Brewer, Jr. In Juvenile Rheumatoid Arthritis. Philadelphia: W.B. Saunders, Co., 1970, pp. 180–222.

51. Rubin, A., Rodda, B.E., Warrick, P. et al. Interactions of aspirin with nonsteroidal antiinflammatory drugs in man. *Arthritis Rheum.* 16:635–45, 1973.

52. Forestier, J. The treatment of rheumatoid arthritis with gold salts injection. *Lancet 1:*441–4, 1932.

53. The Research Subcommittee of the Empire Rheumatism Council. Gold therapy in rheumatoid arthritis final report of a multicenter controlled trial. *Ann Rheum Dis.* 20:315–33, 1961.

54. Edstöm, G., and Gedda, P.O. Clinical prognosis of rheumatoid arthritis in children. *Acta Rheum Scand.* 3:129–53, 1957.

55. Sairanen, E., and Laaksonen, A.-L. The toxicity of gold therapy in children suffering from rheumatoid arthritis. *Ann Paediat Fenn.* 8:105–9, 1962.

56. Sairanen, E., and Laaksonen, A.-L. The results of gold therapy in juvenile rheumatoid arthritis. *Ann Paediat Fenn.* 10:274–9, 1964.

204

57. Hanson, V., Hicks, R., and Kornreich, H. Gold therapy in the treatment of juvenile rheumatoid arthritis. In *Eighth International Congress of Pediatrics*. Neunkirchen, Austria: F. Feilhaur, 1971, pp. 169–74.

58. Levinson, J.E., and Balz, G.P. Gold therapy. *Arthritis Rheum.* 20 (suppl):531–5, 1977.

59. Persellin, R.H., Hess, E.V., and Ziff, M. Effect of a gold salt on the immune response. *Arthritis Rheum.* 10:99–106, 1967.

60. Zutshi, D.W., Ansell, B.M., Bywaters, E.G.L. et al. FII Haemagglutination test for serum antigammaglobulin factor in Still's disease. *Ann Rheum Dis.* 28:541–6, 1969.

61. Jessop, J.D., Vernon-Roberts, B., and Harris, J. Effects of gold salts and prednisolone on inflammatory cells. I. Phagocytic activity of macrophages and polymorphs in inflammatory exudates studied by a "skin window" technique in rheumatoid and control patients. *Ann Rheum Dis.* 32:294–300, 1973.

62. Vernon-Roberts, B., Jessop, J.D., and Dore, J.L. Effects of gold salts and prednisolone on inflammatory cells. II. Suppression of inflammation and phagocytosis in the rat. *Ann Rheum Dis.* 32:301–7, 1973.

63. Vernon-Roberts, B., Dore, J.L., Jessop, J.D., and Henderson, W.J. Selective concentration and localization of gold in macrophages of synovial and other tissues during and after chrysotherapy in rheumatoid patients. *Ann Rheum Dis.* 35:477–86, 1976.

64. Ennis, R.S., Granda, J.L., and Posner, A.S. Effect of gold salts and other drugs on the release and activity of lysosomal hydrolases. *Arthritis Rheum.* 11:756–64, 1968.

65. Perper, R.J., and Oronsky, A.L. Enzyme release from human leukocytes and degradation of cartilage matrix. *Arthritis Rheum.* 17:47–55, 1974.

66. Mascarenhas, B.R., Cranda, J.L., and Freyberg, R.H. Gold metabolism in patients with rheumatoid arthritis treated with gold compounds—reinvestigated. *Arthritis Rheum.* 15:391–402, 1972.

67. Freyberg, R.J., (Revised by) Ziff, M., and Baum, J. Gold therapy for rheumatoid arthritis. Edited by J.L. Hollander and J.J. McCarty, Jr. In *Arthritis and Allied Conditions*. 8th ed. Philadelphia: Lea and Febiger, 1972, pp. 455–82.

68. Anttila, R., and Laaksonen, A.-L. Renal disease in juvenile rheumatoid arthritis. *Acta Rheum Scand.* 15:99–111, 1969.

69. Lorber, A., Atkins, C.J., Chang, C.C. et al. Monitoring serum gold values to improve chrysotherapy in rheumatoid arthritis. *Ann Rheum Dis.* 32:133–9, 1973.

70. Gottlieb, N.L., Smith, P.M., and Smith, E.M. Pharmacodynamics of [197]Au and [195]Au labeled aurothiomalate in blood. *Arthritis Rheum.* 17:171–83, 1974.

71. Sigler, J.W., Bluhm, G.B., Duncan, H. et al. Gold salts in the treatment of rheumatoid arthritis: a double-blind study. *Ann Intern Med.* 80:21–6, 1974.

72. Penneys, N.S., Ackerman, A.B., and Gottlieb, N.L. Gold dermatitis: a clinical and histopathological study. *Arch Dermatol.* 109:372–6, 1974.

73. Davis, P., Ezeoke, A., Munro, J. et al. Immunological studies on the mechanism of gold hypersensitivity reactions. *Br Med J.* 3:676–8, 1973.

74. Howell, A., Gumpel, J.M., and Watts, R.W.E. Depression of bone marrow colony formation in gold-induced neutropenia. *Br Med J.* 1:432–4, 1975.

75. Stavem, P., Stromme, J., and Bull, O. Immunological studies in a case of gold salt-induced thrombocytopenia. *Scand J Haematol.* 5:271–7, 1968.

76. Thompson, D.M., Pegelow, C.H., Singsen, B.H. et al. Neutropenia associated with chrysotherapy for juvenile rheumatoid arthritis. *J Pediatr.* (In press) 1978.

77. England, J.M., and Smith, D.S. Gold-induced thrombocytopenia and response to dimercaprol. *Br Med J.* 2:748–9, 1972.

78. Törnroth, T., and Skrifvars, B. Gold nephropathy prototype of membranous glomerulonephritis. *Am J Pathol.* 75:573–84, 1974.

79. Page, F. Treatment of lupus erythematosus with Mepacrine. *Lancet* 2:755–8, 1951.

80. Freedman, A., and Bach, F. Mepacrine and rheumatoid arthritis. *Lancet* 2:321–2, 1952.

81. Dubois, E.L., editor. *Lupus Erythematosus.* 2nd ed. Los Angeles: University of Southern California Press, 1974, pp. 541–54.

82. Mackenzie, A.H. An appraisal of chloroquine. *Arthritis Rheum.* 13:280–91, 1970.

83. Weissmann, G. Lysosomes and joint disease. *Arthritis Rheum.* 9:834–40, 1966.

84. Ward, P.A. The chemosuppression of chemotasis. *J Exp Med.* 24:209–25, 1966.

85. Mackenzie, A.J., and Scherbel, A.L. A decade of chloroquine maintenance therapy: rate of administration governs incidence of retinopathy, abstracted. *Arthritis Rheum.* 11:496, 1968.

86. Markowitz, H.A., and McGinley, J.M. Cloroquine poisoning in a child. *JAMA.* 189:950–1, 1964.

87. Hamilton, E.B.D., and Scott, J.T. Hydroxychloroquine sulfate ("Plaquenil") in treatment of rheumatoid arthritis. *Arthritis Rheum.* 5:502–12, 1962.

88. Ansell, B.M. Principles in the medical treatment of Still's disease. Edited by M.I.V. Jayson. In *Still's Disease: Juvenile Chronic Polyarthritis.* London: Academic Press, 1976, p. 225.

89. Laaksonen, A.-L., Koskiahde, V., and Juva, K. Dosage of antimalarial drugs for children with juvenile rheumatoid arthritis and systemic lupus erythematosus. *Scand J Rheumatol.* 3:103–8, 1974.

90. Jaffe, I.A. Rheumatoid arthritis with arteritis. Report of a case treated with penicillamine. *Ann Int Med.* 61:556–62, 1964.

91. The Multicenter Trial Group. Controlled trial of d(-) penicillamine in severe rheumatoid arthritis. *Lancet* 1:275–80, 1973.

92. Zuckner, J., Ramsey, R.H., Dorner, R.W., and Gantner, G.E. d-penicillamine in rheumatoid arthritis. *Arthritis Rheum.* 13:131–8, 1970.

93. Bluestone, R., and Goldberg, L.S. Effect of d-penicillamine on serum immunoglobulins and rheumatoid factor. *Ann Rheum Dis.* 32:50–62, 1973.

94. Jaffe, I.A. The treatment of rheumatoid arthritis and necrotizing vasculitis with penicillamine. *Arthritis Rheum.* 13:436–43, 1970.

95. Moynahan, E.F. d(-) penicillamine in morphea (localized scleroderma). *Lancet* 1:428–9, 1973.

96. Harris, E.D., and Sjoerdsma, A. Effect of penicillamine on human collagen and its possible application to treatment of scleroderma. *Lancet* 2:996–9, 1966.

206

97. Ansell, B., and Hall, M.A. Penicillamine. *Arthritis Rheum.* 20 (suppl):536, 1977.

98. Hench, P.S. The potential reversibility of rheumatoid arthritis. *Mayo Clin Proc.* 24:167–78, 1949.

99. Schlesinger, B.E., Forsyth, C.C., White, R.H.R. et al. Observations on the clinical course and treatment of one hundred cases of Still's disease. *Arch Dis Child.* 36:65–76, 1961.

100. Ansell, B.M., Bywaters, E.G.L., and Isdale, I.C. Comparison of cortisone and aspirin in treatment of juvenile rheumatoid arthritis. *Br Med J.* 1:1075–7, 1956.

101. Good, R.A., Vernier, R.L., and Smith, R.T. Serious untoward reactions to therapy with cortisone and adrenocorticotropin in pediatric practice (Part 1). *Pediatrics.* 19:95–118, 1957.

102. Bernstein, B., Stobie, D., Singsen, B.H. et al. Growth retardation in juvenile rheumatoid arthritis (JRA). *Arthritis Rheum.* 20 (suppl):212–16, 1977.

103. Van Metre, T.E., Niermann, W.A., and Rosen, L.J. A comparison of the growth suppressive effect of cortisone, prednisone, and other adrenal cortical hormones. *J Allergy.* 31:531, 1960.

104. Schaller, J.G. Corticosteroids in juvenile rheumatoid arthritis. *Arthritis Rheum.* 20 (suppl):537–43, 1977.

105. Good, T.A., Benton, J.W., and Kelley, V.C. Symptomatology resulting from withdrawal of steroid hormone therapy. *Arthritis Rheum.* 2:299–321, 1959.

106. Baum, J., and Gutowska, G. Death in juvenile rheumatoid arthritis. *Arthritis Rheum.* 20 (suppl):253–5, 1977.

107. Bernstein, B., Takahashi, M., and Hanson, V. Cardiac involvement in juvenile rheumatoid arthritis. *J Pediatr.* 85:313–17, 1974.

108. Fürst, C., Smiley, W.K., and Ansell, B.M. Steroid cataract. *Ann Rheum Dis.* 25:364–8, 1966.

109. MacGregor, R.R., Sheagren, J.N., Lipsett, M.B. et al. Alternate-day prednisone therapy. *N Engl J Med.* 280:1427–31, 1969.

110. Soyka, L.F. Alternate-day corticosteroid therapy. *Adv Pediatr.* 19:47–70, 1972.

111. Ansell, B.M., and Bywaters, E.G.L. Alternate-day corticosteroid therapy in juvenile chronic polyarthritis. *J Rheumatol.* 1:176–86, 1974.

112. Zutshi, D.W., Friedman, M., and Ansell, B.M. Corticotrophin therapy in juvenile chronic polyarthritis (Still's disease) and effect on growth. *Arch Dis Child.* 46:584–93, 1971.

113. Chylack, L.T., Jr. The ocular manifestations of juvenile rheumatoid arthritis. *Arthritis Rheum.* 20 (suppl):217–23, 1977.

114. Black, R.L., O'Brien, W.M., Van Scott, E.J. et al. Methotrexate therapy in psoriatic arthritis: double-blind study on 21 patients. *JAMA.* 189:743–7, 1964.

115. Sokoloff, M.C., Goldberg, L.S., and Pearson, C.M. Treatment of corticosteroid resistant polymyositis with methotrexate. *Lancet 1*:14–16, 1971.

116. Calabresi, P., and Parks, R.E., Jr. Alkylating agents, antimetabolites, hormones, and other antiproliferative agents. Edited by L.S. Goodman and A. Gilman. In *The Pharmacological Basis of Therapeutics.* 4th ed. New York: The MacMillan Company, 1970, pp. 1348–95.

117. Elion, G.B. Biochemistry and pharmacology of purine analogs. *Proc Soc Exp Biol.* 26:898–904, 1967.

118. Hollister, J.R. Immunosuppressant therapy of juvenile rheumatoid arthritis. *Arthritis Rheum.* 20 (suppl):544–7, 1977.

119. Cooperative Clinics Committee of the American Rheumatism Association. A controlled trial of cyclophosphamide in rheumatoid arthritis. *N Engl J Med.* 283:883–9, 1970.

120. De Sèze, S., Bédoiseau, M., DeBeyre, N., and Kahn, M.F. Resultats de la therapeutique à visée immunodépressive chez 40 malades atteints de polyarthrite rheumatöide grave. *Sem Hôp Paris.* 43:3084–91, 1967.

121. Godfrey, W.A., Epstein, W.V., O'Connor, G.R. et al. The use of chlorambucil in intractable idiopathic uveitis. *Am J Ophthalmol.* 78:415–28, 1974.

122. Rudd, P., Fries, J.F., and Epstein, W.V. Irreversible bone marrow failure with chlorambucil. *J Rheumatol.* 2:421–9, 1975.

123. Skinner, M.D., and Schwartz, R.S. Immunosuppressive therapy. Part 2. *N Engl J Med.* 287:281–6, 1972.

124. Snaith, M.L., Holt, J.M., Oliver, D.O. et al. Treatment of patients with systemic lupus erythematosus, including nephritis, with chlorambucil. *Br Med J.* 2:197–201, 1973.

125. Urowitz, M.B., Gordon, D.A., Smythe, H.A. et al. Azathioprine in rheumatoid arthritis. A double-blind, cross-over study. *Arthritis Rheum.* 16:411–18, 1973.

126. Hunter, T., Urowitz, M.B., Gordon, D.A. et al. Azathioprine in rheumatoid arthritis. A long-term follow-up study. *Arthritis Rheum.* 18:15–20, 1975.

127. Dale, I. The treatment of juvenile rheumatoid arthritis with azathioprine. *Scand J Rheumatol.* 1:125–7, 1972.

128. Fahey, J.L. Cancer in the immunosuppressed patient. *Ann Intern Med.* 75:310–12, 1971.

15 Physical Measures in the Treatment of Juvenile Rheumatoid Arthritis

William H. Donovan

The intent of this chapter is to provide a rational approach to the prescription of splints, heat, therapeutic exercises and other physical measures for the patient with JRA. Examples are given of certain physical measures found by the author to be beneficial, but there is no intent to imply that omitted items are not useful or that those mentioned should be used exclusively. No attempt will be made to compare the merits of physical against surgical methods of treatment or to suggest when the former should end and the latter begin.

Fundamentally one must remember that juvenile rheumatoid arthritis (JRA) is a group of syndromes rather than a single entity,[1] and that prior to prescribing any physical treatments one should ask the following medical and psychosocial questions about the disease, the patient and the parents. Medical: (1) What form of JRA does the patient have; (2) what is the observed and expected degree of local and systemic disease activity; (3) what critical functions in the child's activities of daily living (eating, dressing, bathing, toileting, transferring, and walking) are impaired; (4) with what kind of deformity(ies) is the child likely to end up? Psychosocial: (1) How intelligent and cooperative are the parents; (2) how well does the child and how well do the parents understand the disease and the need for comprehensive medical management; (3) how has the disease interfered with normal psychologic growth of the child at home and school; (4) how has it interfered with family function and how are the parents coping; (5) how much initiative has been taken to make architectural modifications of the home and school environment for the more severely disabled child; (6) how close does the family live to a treatment facility and is transportation thereto available; and (7) will the family need financial assistance? When these factors are known, the physician will be able to make maximum use of the services of allied health professions, such as physical therapists, occupational therapists and social workers. In turn he or she will have a better understanding of how and why the prescribed treatment is succeeding or failing.

Prescribing physical measures is not as simple as prescribing medication for the arthritic or any other child with a disability. In some localities services are not readily available and many insurance companies exclude payment for them. Agencies such as Washington state's Crippled Children's Services and Public Assistance often authorize payment only after they receive a request for treatment from the physician in writing and insist on screening for financial eligibility which inevitably creates delays in initiating treatment. Some school systems provide therapy services, but only when school is in session. In most instances therefore, the parents must be trained to carry out and to supervise the therapy on a daily basis. This may be inconvenient and compliance will often be poor, but attention to these facts is necessary if the physician wishes to be sure the patient receives the physical measures prescribed.[2]

The therapeutic goals for which these measures are employed usually will include: (1) reducing pain and inflammation, (2) minimizing joint destruction and deformity, (3) maintaining or improving range of motion and function as much as possible, (4) maintaining or improving muscle strength for adequate protection of the involved joints, and (5) providing the patient with the necessary treatment, equipment, and information so the first four goals can be reached and so the family can make as optimal an adjustment as possible if permanent disability does develop.

SPLINTING

When prescribing splints the physician should have some knowledge not only of the activity of the disease within the joint but also the direction in which the deformity is likely to develop and the force necessary to prevent it or produce correction. While these forces in arthritis are generally not as great as those encountered when treating such conditions as spasticity they can be considerable, and attention must be paid to the skin where the force is concentrated. If the skin remains hyperemic after wearing the splint for more than 15 minutes or if the child complains of pain at a specific pressure point the splint should be modified so the restraining or correcting force can be distributed over a wider area. The splint must be comfortable enough to be tolerated for a protracted period of time. It has been shown that a low stretching force can be effective in distending collagenous tissue, particularly if heat is applied and the tissue temperature raised, but a long duration of treatment is required.[3]

Choice of Splint

The choice of splints will largely depend on the activity of the disease[4] (Table 1).

When the joint is acutely inflamed and even slight movement is painful maximum rest or immobilization of the joint and the tendons crossing it should be provided. For example for active disease in the wrist, both the wrist and metacarpophalangeal and interphalangeal joints should be immobilized since the tendons activating the distal joints cross the wrist and may be involved. A *resting splint* (Figure 1) will reduce all forces to which the joint may be subjected, both externally and by the effects of muscle contraction. Immobilization in this way allows optimal reduction of inflammation and pain.[5]

As soon as intense pain is controlled and guarding is reduced *functional splints* which rest the affected joint, but not those distal to it, can be used. For some joints, e.g., the knee and elbow, functional and resting splints are not different, but for the wrist and ankle functional splints permit movement of the distal joints. This freedom is especially important when the wrist is immobilized, for if the fingers can move numerous daily activities can still be performed and the splint will be much more easily accepted by the child. When finger joints alone must be splinted, the plastic or metal finger splints described by Bennett for older children are preferred[6] (Figure 2).

When disease has become further controlled and the child can tolerate the discomfort *corrective splints* can be used (Figure 3). Age and ability of the child and parents to endure should be considered before prescribing corrective splints because each new setting will cause an increase in discomfort. The joint is placed in the maximally tolerated position in the desired direction and secured in that position until range improves. Then the setting is advanced. Serial plaster

Table 1
Splinting

Disease Activity	Purpose of Splint	When Splint Applied	Desirable Characteristics of Splint
Acute inflammatory episodes.	a) Provide joint rest.	a) 24 hrs/day until inflammatory response improves.	a) Set in "position of function" or as close to optimum position as pain will allow.
	b) Reduce inflammation.	b) Remove b.i.d. for gentle active assistive range of motion.	b) Immobilize affected joint(s) plus tendons crossing the joint which activate other joints.
			c) Removable: Easy to apply and remove.
Chronically active — likely to flare frequently.	a) Prevent deformities.	a) Each night for as long as tolerated.	a) Set in "position of function" or as close to optimum position as possible.
	b) Improve function.	b) During activities. Nonsplinted joints are free to function.	b) Removable: Easy to apply and remove.
			c) Easily modified to accomodate a decrease in deformity.
			d) Immobilize affected joint, leaving other joints free.

| Chronic-controlled. | Increase range of motion, reduce deformity.

N.B. Some children will not be able to tolerate initial discomfort of this type of splint. | Each night for as long as tolerated. | a) Set in position of maximum attainable range.
b) Removable.
c) Can be either:
dynamic-continuous tension via rubber bands or springs (N.B. axis of splint must match anatomical axis)

OR

static-fixed position. Regularly scheduled changes to allow for the increase in range of motion should be made. |

214

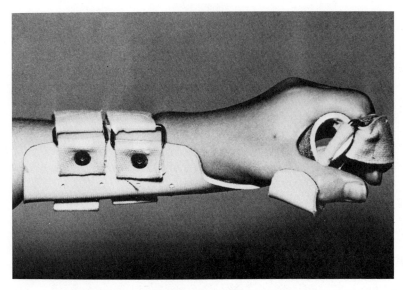

Figure 1. Resting splint for wrist positioned at 20° dorsiflexion. MP and IP joints also immobilized by distal strap at optimal angles to preserve function.

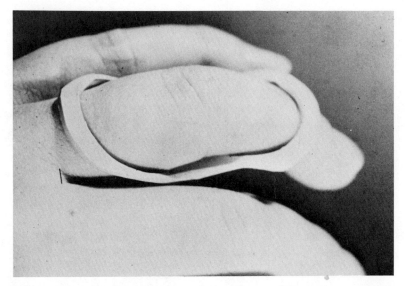

Figure 2. Ring splint which prevents hyperextension of PIP joint as used in child developing swan neck deformities as result of chronic PIP joint disease.

casting is not advocated in JRA since joints have a tendency to ankylose, and carrying out a daily range of motion is important. Other disadvantages of plaster casting include the expense of frequent cast changes and the necessity for patients to return just for this purpose. *Moldable plastics* such as Warm N Form, Kay Splinting and Orthoplast are preferable, not only for corrective splints but for resting and functional splints because they permit a new setting when range improves, and are removable so that daily range of motion can be performed.

Position of Function

Every effort is made to restore the joint to its position of function or most useful position which varies with each joint. The ankle or tibiotalar joint should be "neutral," that is, with the foot flat on the floor the

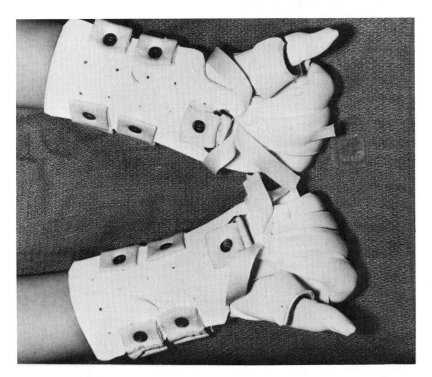

Figure 3. Corrective splints on child with quiescent disease to increase MP and IP flexion. Cotton strips are sewn to fingertips of gloves and individually tightened under D-clasp. Splint formerly used as functional splint.

tibia should be inclined 7° to 10° anteriorly from the vertical when viewed from the side. Either a splint or an ankle-foot orthosis is suitable. The preferred position for the knee is as close to full extension as pain and swelling will permit since the forces acting on the knee during weight-bearing are least in this position. However, as it is important to have close to 90° of flexion at the knee for sitting, persistent active or gentle active assistive range-of-motion exercises are necessary.

Metacarpophalangeal joints have a tendency to ankylose in extension in JRA. Forty-five degrees of flexion of the index and third MP joints and slightly more in the fourth and fifth MP joints should be maintained. Loss of flexion range in these joints is more disabling than loss of extension.[7] For the wrist, 15° to 20° of dorsiflexion is preferred as this position affords the least handicap if the wrist fuses. Although some activities in this position are difficult, e.g., toileting and buttoning, it is the most acceptable compromise for most activities of daily living, particularly if the range of motion at the shoulder is normal. No one position is optimal for the elbow, because the purpose of this joint is the "breaking" of the upper extremity to permit reach and return of objects and to allow the hand to operate close and far from the body. Nevertheless, when splinting the elbow is necessary, 90° of flexion has proven to be the most satisfactory compromise. Every effort should be made using range-of-motion exercises to preserve as much movement as possible in flexion and extension and in pronation and supination.

Splinting the hip or shoulder is not practical. Bed positioning, such as lying in the prone position, and skin traction can be used to maintain the desired position of the hip. Full extension and 90° of flexion should be preserved if at all possible. If fusion of the joint occurs, 20° of flexion (or 160° extension) is the least disabling, as sitting can be tolerated if sufficient flexion of the lumbar spine is present and standing is possible with the aid of crutches. The shoulder can be splinted in a sling when the symptoms are acute and immobilization is needed. However, the sling should be removed in bed and the arm positioned at about 70° of abduction with a pillow. When pain subsides the sling should be discarded and range-of-motion exercises pursued intensively since the shoulder capsule has a marked tendency to develop contractures. If the glenohumeral articulation alone is involved, some substitution for motion can be gained by movement of the scapula, especially if the sternoclavicular and acromioclavicular joints are uninvolved. Frequently restricted range at the glenohumeral joint is less disabling than anticipated, and if 90° of flexion, abduction, and external rotation are maintained at the shoulder, most activities of daily living can be performed.

The neck can be partially immobilized at roughly 30° of flexion with a soft collar. If more rigid immobilization is needed a four poster type brace or Somi brace can be used. When symptoms subside the collar or brace should be gradually discontinued. If subluxation of the atlantoaxial joint occurs, as it can in acute stages, it is advisable to wear cervical protection when involved in any activity in which sudden unpredictable force to the neck may occur, e.g., when riding in an automobile. Immobilization or bracing of the thoracic and/or lumbar spine is generally not necessary except when wedge compression fractures of the vertebral bodies are encountered. This is generally a complication of steroid therapy, (Figures 4 and 5) and virtually never associated with spinal cord dysfunction but can lead to a progressive kyphotic deformity. Treatment consists of bed-rest on a firm surface until pain subsides followed by progressive weight-bearing while maintaining immobilization in an extension brace.

Duration of Application

Splints should be worn all day when joints are acutely inflamed except for removal twice daily for range-of-motion exercises. This allows the beneficial effects of immobilization to reduce inflammation[5] and movement to decrease the chances of contracture and ankylosis. Splints should be worn even if patients are in bed all day since movements and positions favoring deformity continue and may be worse for some joints. Controversy still remains as to whether complete immobilization will in fact lead to fusion or irreversible ankylosis. Complete immobilization for four weeks has been shown to produce neither permanent contractures nor significant gains in range of motion in adult rheumatoid arthritis, but there is evidence to support the efficacy of daily range-of-motion exercises for patients with JRA even when active inflammation is present.[8-11] After acute inflammation has subsided functional splints are worn at night and for specified times during the day, usually one-half to one hour twice a day, but free movement of the joint is allowed the rest of the day. The actual time spent in the splint should be individually tailored to each child keeping in mind those factors mentioned above. If the child is rewarded for adherence to this schedule splint-wearing is less of a problem for all concerned. When a decrease in the activity of the disease permits the use of corrective splints, they should be worn as long as possible, except for exercise periods. In the cases of children who do not tolerate the sustained static stretch of corrective splints even when the disease is well

218

controlled, functional splints should be continued in the hope that exercises alone will bring improvement in range of motion. Those who can tolerate corrective splints may use either dynamic or static splints. Dynamic splints used primarily on wrists and fingers, maintain tension via springs or rubber bands that can be added or subtracted depending upon the goals, the disease activity, and the patient's tolerance. They often meet with poor acceptance by young children and so are rarely used. Static splints have to be changed periodically, as indicated above, but are more suitable for the pediatric population.

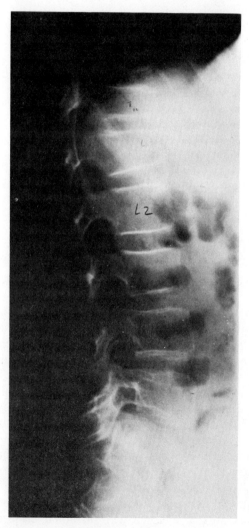

Figure 4. Lumbar spine roentgenograph of child with systemic polyarticular JRA treated with steroids for 18 months. Note wedging of T12 and L1.

Special Considerations

Some joints require particular attention when splinted, the foremost example being the knee. Splinting or stretching of the knee may result in posterior subluxation of the tibia,[12] which is apt to occur if wedging plaster casts or other splints that attempt to correct flexion contractures with only a hinge are used. Functional and corrective splints should fit from upper thigh to ankle and be well molded so an anteriorly

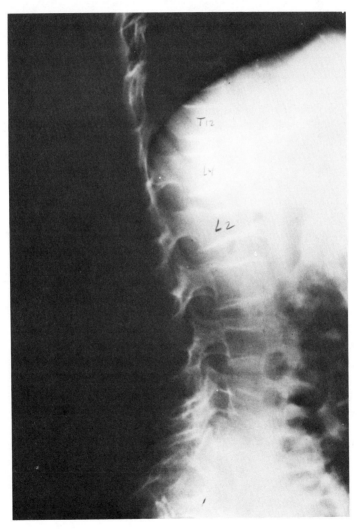

Figure 5. Lumbar spine roentgenograph of same patient taken 1 month later. Patient experienced sudden onset of back pain and tenderness over L2 after simply rising from wheelchair to standing position.

directed force is maintained against the proximal tibia. The circular knee strap should be just proximal to the place where the patella lies in full extension. When joint deformities in the lower extremities exist, walking may increase the deformity. This is especially important in the knee due to the large forces created if one walks with the joint in flexed position. No formula is available to relate a child's weight to that flexion-contracture angle beyond which the deformity is likely to increase if weight-bearing is permitted, however, it would seem wise to consider limiting walking in children who lack more than 15° to full extension.

Splinting of the feet may best be accomplished by form-fitting insoles made of soft moldable material such as Plastazote which distribute weight-bearing more evenly over the entire foot and may be sufficient to relieve metatarsalgia. Occasionally metatarsal bars on the outside of the shoe will be necessary to transfer the force of body weight against the floor from the metatarsal heads to the plantar arch. Before using them, however, one should be sure the articulations in the area of the arch are pain-free and can absorb the increased pressure.

In some instances, particularly the pauciarticular form of JRA involving one knee, increased leg length may be noted on the affected side. Shoe lifts added to heel and sole of the unaffected side are usually prescribed to reduce the energy cost of walking if the difference exceeds 1 cm. The forces on the affected knee due to flexion throughout the gait cycle are reduced and back pain from an uneven pelvis is averted.

HEAT

It is generally accepted that heat treatments are useful adjuncts in the management of rheumatoid arthritis. Table 2 outlines a suggested approach to thermotherapy. Only superficial heat administered by contact with warm water, towels, or packs, or less often infrared radiation, should be used during the acute or chronically active stages, to promote analgesia and muscle relaxation, rather than to heat the joint. Heat treatments generally last at least 20 to 30 minutes, the temperature in hydrotherapy varying with the extent of body surface submerged; up to 110° F for an extremity and 90 to 95° F for the whole body.[13] Such hot baths are useful in relieving morning stiffness and range-of-motion exercise is made easier because of the reduction of pain and guarding. Contrast baths, i.e., alternating hot and cool water, are frequently impractical for small children but can be of benefit in relieving morning stiffness in older children. Cold has been reported to be of symptomatic benefit to patients with adult RA,[14] but no reports of its effectiveness in children are available. It should be used only locally over the affected joint and the muscles that activate it, and only if it enhances pain relief.

Paraffin baths are useful for the treatment of wrists and fingers in some cases if the technique of dipping the hand in and out eight to ten times is followed. However, unless one of the newer thermostatically controlled units is used the work involved in the preparation of the paraffin outweighs the benefits and many parents will not comply. In addition, small children are often afraid of placing their hands in the paraffin.

Table 2
An Approach to Thermotherapy

Disease Activity	Physical Modalities Used
Acute Inflammatory Episodes	Superficial heat a) general: water, 90°–98°F (tank, pool, tub) b) local: water, 90°–98°F Superficial cold a) local only *Purpose:* increase pain threshold
Chronically active Likely to reflare	Superficial Heat a) general: water, 90°–98°F (tank, pool, tub) b) local: water, 95°–104°F, paraffin Massage — gentle stroking of muscles (if painful) which activate the joint. Joint itself not massaged *Purpose:* increase pain threshold Traction a) skin traction applied at night and/or while napping (hip) *Purpose:* static stretch preserve range of motion some pain relief
Chronic-controlled	Superficial Heat a) general: water, 90°–98° F (tank, pool, tub) b) local: water, 95°–104°F, paraffin *Purpose:* increase pain threshold Deep Heat a) local only ultrasound, shortwave or microwave diathermy *Purpose:* increase temperature of connective tissue around joint which raises pain threshold, increases collagen elasticity and allows improved response to static stretch Traction a) skin traction applied at night and/or while napping (hip) *Purpose:* static stretch increase range of motion

Diathermy machines warm the deeper structures more than the skin. Shortwave and microwave diathermy at available wave lengths produce maximum temperatures only a few centimeters below the skin surface. Ultrasound, which has the deepest penetration, is the only effective means of heating joints covered by large amounts of soft tissue, e.g., the hip, and is the only safe method of deep heating of joints which contain metal implants.[13] However, it should be used only if all acute inflammatory signs have subsided and only the residua remain, i.e., scarring and contractures, because the physiologic responses to deep heat at temperatures of 107° to 109° F consist of an increase in blood flow and vasodilation, an increase in tissue metabolism, and a decrease in tissue pH, and thus are similar to some of the acute inflammatory responses from rheumatoid arthritis itself. Although tissue damage could result from deep heating during the acute phase the connective tissue around the joint can be raised to these temperatures and the tissues can tolerate it when acute synovitis has subsided.[13] In addition to raising the pain threshold the deep heat facilitates elongation of the connective tissue, and for this reason diathermy treatment should be combined with slow static stretching.[3]

Recognized contraindications for all forms of heat treatments are the presence of impaired sensation of the skin over the affected joint, decreased circulation in the affected limb, and the presence of a coagulation defect.[9]

EXERCISE

Therapeutic exercises generally employed in the treatment of JRA consist of active and active assistive range of motion, isometric strengthening contractions, and general conditioning (Table 3) preferably performed twice a day.[11]

Active and Active Assistive Range-of-Motion Exercise

Active assistive range-of-motion exercise consists of the patient moving the affected joint within a pain-free range while the therapist or parent gently guides it further if possible. This permits movement of the joint, its capsule, and adjoining tendons, but avoids much of the compressive forces that occur with active movement. When inflammation has begun to subside active assistive motion is generally employed to coax the joint slowly into the extremes where pain is felt. It is held just under this point for a fixed count, usually between five and ten seconds and is repeated five to ten times as tolerated.

Most clinicians believe that repeated movement of an acutely inflamed joint will aggravate the inflammation. This has been shown to be true in experimental arthritides.[15] Since objective limits are unknown, pain is generally the best guideline for determining how many times a joint should be ranged and how long it should be held at the extremes of range when the inflammation has subsided. Swezey has suggested that if pain increases after one session of exercise and persists for more than two hours, repetitions and/or duration of time in extremes of range should be reduced during the next session.[9]

Table 3
An Approach to Exercise

Disease Activity	Type of Therapeutic Exercise
Acute Inflammatory Episodes	Active Assistive Range of Motion a) patient moves joint actively as far as possible b) therapist moves joint passively to (maximum) limits Isometric strengthening a) in desired joint position, if possible b) emphasis on antigravity muscles c) 6 seconds hold 1–2 seconds relax, repeat d) can be done in splint General conditioning a) pool

Chronically active Likely to reflare	Active Assistive Range of Motion
	a) patient moves joint actively as far as possible
	b) therapist moves joint passively to maximum limits
	   (with mild terminal stretch if tolerated)
	             OR
	patient uses positioning of body weight to provide passive assist and stretch
	Active Range of Motion
	Isometric strengthening
	General conditioning
	a) pool
	N.B. progressive resistive and other isotonic exercises to be avoided

Chronic-controlled	Active Range of Motion (no resistance) if patient can carry the joint to limits of passive range
	Active Assistive Range of Motion if patient cannot
	Isometric strengthening
	General conditioning
	   a) pool
	   b) bicycle/tricycle
	   c) Marx "Big Wheel"

Since intensity of symptoms and tolerance for exercise may vary with time of day, medication schedule (particularly if alternate-day steroids are prescribed), and the availability of heat, one should be sure conditions are optimal before advising the therapist or parents to carry out range-of-motion exercises.

The older patient, using his own body weight or other extremity, can perform active assistive exercises himself. For example by controlling his body weight and leaning against a wall or desk with the palms against the surface, he can supply a gentle stretch of the wrist joint into dorsiflexion.

Isometric Strengthening

There is no reason to strengthen muscles that activate the arthritic joint beyond the point where they can adequately protect its cartilage and restraining ligaments from undue force. Under experimental conditions it has been shown that to insure a normal muscle's gain in strength it should be taken to the point of fatigue, but this may not be possible in the arthritic patient because pain may intervene.[16] Therefore strengthening exercises may do no more than retard disuse atrophy during acute phases of disease. Since repeated movement especially against resistance may aggravate the arthritis it is advisable to use isometric exercises in which muscles that activate the arthritic joint contract but the joint does not move. Isometrics can be performed by having the patient contract both the agonist (e.g., quadriceps) and antagonist (e.g., hamstrings) simultaneously or by holding the limb segment in a fixed position against resistance (e.g., holding the knee extended against gravity while the thigh is supported). Children over four years of age can usually carry out a series of isometric contractions or sets held to the count of six and repeated up to 10 to 20 times, at the extremes of active range; younger children need a game activity to accomplish the same objective. This technique can maintain or improve muscle strength providing sufficient force can be generated and can assist in the achievement of increased range of motion.[17] Patients are begun on isometrics even during acute flare-ups. They are instructed to continue to perform the sets twice daily, in a splint or without during all phases of disease activity, but are told *not* to perform any exercise that loads or places undue forces across an involved joint such as is done in lifting weights, squeezing a rubber ball, and other progressive resistive exercises at any time. Such isotonic exercises, i.e., those in which muscle contraction moves the joint against resistance, can hasten deformity and ligamentous disruption since the forces are dissipated in abnormal directions.

General Conditioning Exercises

There is no substitute for pool activities, such as swimming, splashing, walking, or games geared to improve range of motion.[18] The buoyant effect of water allows larger weight-bearing joints to be moved with little force. Walking can be painless in water since body weight passing through the joint is negligible if a child is submerged to his or her shoulders and as the symptoms improve he or she can move into gradually shallower water. Water can also provide gentle resistance to any movement when the hydraulic effect is utilized, i.e., the faster the limb segment is moved, the greater the resistance and vice versa. If the temperature of the water is 90° F or higher, an analgesic effect can also be expected. Thirty to 60 minutes of pool activities daily is extremely helpful. Every effort must be made to help children overcome fear of water. Some do better in pool therapy with parents present, but most small children perform better without them, at least initially.

If walking is painful, children with arthritis of weight-bearing joints are encouraged to use a tricycle or "Big Wheel." These permit activity of the affected joints and muscles and provide mobility. These devices are generally more suitable for the younger arthritic child than ambulatory aids such as crutches, walkerettes, and canes, and wheelchairs which are preferable for older children. Games that involve the use of the appropriate joints can provide a general active range of motion and can be demonstrated to the parents and child by a physical or occupational therapist. Parents should be instructed to allow the patient to do as much for himself or herself as possible because even tasks such as dressing and bathing constitute therapeutic range of motion.

BRACING

There is generally little need for braces for arthritics since they are not used to *correct* deformities. Braces are generally utilized to substitute for muscle power, maintain joint stability and alignment, and in some cases provide for protection against weight-bearing. None of these three purposes is applicable to the child with JRA except rare instances when bracing of an ankle or knee will maintain joint stability and yet permit more mobility than is allowed by splints.[11]

REST

Controversy still surrounds the subject of rest for the arthritic. No study has yet been done in children which is comparable to that undertaken with adults which found no significant difference between rested and nonrested hospitalized populations.[19] Children will most often limit their own activity when the disease is active so no rules of thumb founded in anything other than clinical experience can be given. Probably a daily routine for a child with JRA ought to include some time for (1) general conditioning, preferably done in water, (2) range-of-motion exercises, and (3) the everyday social and family activities in which normal children of the same age engage. An afternoon nap can be interwoven particularly if it is age-appropriate and if the child welcomes it. However, to enforce more than one or two hours of rest when the child is not fatigued seems pointless and can be a source of persistent parent-child friction. Since there are many other aspects to the daily routine that can act as focuses of friction it would seem that unwelcome mandatory rest need not be an additional one.

REFERENCES

1. Schaller, J., and Wedgwood, R.J. Juvenile rheumatoid arthritis: a review. *Pediatrics.* 50:940–53, 1972.
2. Moon, M.H., Moon, B.A.M., and Black, W.A.M. Compliancy in splint-wearing behavior of patients with rheumatoid arthritis. *NZ Med J.* 83:360–5, 1976.
3. Warren, C.G., Lehmann, J.F., and Koblanski, J.N. Elongation of rat tail tendon: effect of load and temperature. *Arch Phys Med Rehabil.* 52:465–75, 1971.
4. Donovan, W.H. Physical measures in the treatment of juvenile rheumatoid arthritis. *Arthritis Rheum.* 20 (suppl):553–7, 1977.
5. Gault, S.J., and Spyker, J.M. Beneficial effect of immobilization of joints in rheumatoid and related arthritides: a splint study using sequential analysis. *Arthritis Rheum.* 12:34–44, 1969.
6. Bennett, R.L. Orthotic devices to prevent deformities of the hand in rheumatoid arthritis. *Arthritis Rheum.* 8:1006–18, 1965.
7. Brewerton, D.A. Hand deformities in rheumatoid disease. *Ann Rheum Dis.* 16:183–97, 1957.
8. Partridge, R.E.H., and Duthie, J.J.R. Controlled trial of the effects of complete immobilization of the joints in rheumatoid arthritis. *Ann Rheum Dis.* 22:91–8, 1963.
9. Swezey, R.L. Essentials of physical management and rehabilitation in arthritis. *Semin Arthritis Rheum.* 3:349–68, 1974.
10. Rhinelander, F.W. The effectiveness of splinting and bracing on rheumatoid arthritis. *Arthritis Rheum.* 2:270–7, 1959.

11. Murray, W.R. Juvenile rheumatoid arthritis. *Curr Pract Orthop Surg.* 6:171–212, 1975.

12. Convery, F.R., and Minteer, M.A. The use of orthoses in the management of rheumatoid arthritis. *Clin Orthop.* 102:118–25, 1974.

13. Lehmann, J.F., Warren, C.G., and Scham, S.M. Therapeutic heat and cold. *Clin Orthop.* 99:207–45, 1974.

14. Kirt, J.A., and Kersley, G.D. Heat and cold in the physical treatment of rheumatoid arthritis of the knee. *Ann Phys Med.* 9:270–4, 1968.

15. Agudelo, C., Schumacher, H.R., and Phelps, P. Effect of exercise on urate crystal induced inflammation in canine joints. *Arthritis Rheum.* 15:609–15, 1972.

16. DeLateur, B.J., Lehmann, J.F., and Giaconi, R. Mechanical work and fatigue: their roles in the development of muscle work capacity. *Arch Phys Med Rehabil.* 57:319–24, 1976.

17. Muller, E.A. Influence of training and of inactivity on muscle strength. *Arch Phys Med Rehabil.* 51:449–56, 1970.

18. Boone, J.E., and Baldwin, J. Juvenile rheumatoid arthritis. *Pediatr Clin North Am.* 21:885–915, 1974.

19. Mills, J.A., Pinals, R.S., Ropes, M.W. et al. Value of bed-rest in patients with rheumatoid arthritis. *N Engl J Med.* 284:453–8, 1971.

16 Surgical Treatment of Juvenile Rheumatoid Arthritis

Lawrence A. Rinsky

With the early diagnosis and appropriate nonsurgical treatment of juvenile rheumatoid arthritis (JRA) most patients never require operative intervention. In several long term studies, the incidence of patients requiring some surgical procedure has varied from less than 10% to over 25% of patients.[1-4] These data may be somewhat skewed by the natural tendency for more seriously involved patients to be treated at arthritis centers. The purpose of this chapter is to define the indications in JRA for which surgical treatment is beneficial, and to explain briefly the rationale for, technique, and results of the specific operative procedures. Synovectomy is discussed in greater detail because it is controversial. There will also be a discussion of those problems common to all surgical procedures in patients with JRA.

Surgery in JRA should not be considered a radical alternative to conservative treatment, but as an adjunct to medical and physical therapy. The orthopedist's most significant role may be that of the physician who orders physical therapy, splinting, etc. These aspects of treatment are covered in Chapter 15.

SOFT TISSUE OPERATIONS

Contracture Release

Prevention of flexion contractures by physical therapy, resting splints, and medical treatment is obviously desirable. However, when the deformity progresses in spite of adequate nonoperative treatment and interferes with function, surgical release should be considered. This is in general less applicable to the upper extremities where there are more compensatory mechanisms available, than in the lower extremities. An ankylosed shoulder, for example, still has 60° of abduction due to scapulothoracic rotation. With surgical release the entire capsular structures are divided on the concave side of the contracture, and the major tendons lengthened as necessary.

This procedure is most useful for the knee and ankle, although occasionally it is used for the hip or wrist. When contractures are released neurovascular structures on the concave side of the joint have to be carefully protected. Flexion contractures of the knee may be treated with skeletal traction using a pin in the tibia and perhaps the femur,[5] however, prolonged traction is not well tolerated by the patient who has many active joints because the enforced bedrest engenders stiffness in other joints.

Tendon and Ligament Reconstruction

Procedures such as correction of swan neck and boutonniere deformities in fingers are for collapsing lax joints but are rarely performed in children. This is probably because joint destruction results in stiffness and ankylosis in JRA rather than in subluxation and laxity as in adult RA.

Synovectomy

Synovectomy is the most intellectually appealing, yet perhaps the most controversial surgical procedure for JRA. The concept of excising the source of the enzymes responsible for the destruction of the joint surfaces makes sense and has many advocates, however, the literature is full of conflicting opinions as to the efficacy of the procedure.[3-14] It was first used in the early 1900s and has waxed and waned in popularity since.[15,16] Most of the recent reports of synovectomy give a favorable impression of the results in properly selected patients but part of the difficulty in evaluating results is due to the highly variable nature of the prognosis in individual patients. Long-term surveys of JRA show at least 35% to 50% of patients have a complete remission and that an additional 25% to 30% are left with only mild functional disability.[4,12,17] Since surgery of a joint destined to recover spontaneously is undesirable, it would be ideal to be able to predict the course of an individual child's disease. Unfortunately this is not possible, however, some facts, assumptions, and opinions are useful in deciding when to operate.

(1) Synovitis does not immediately cause joint destruction. In most cases it can be controlled medically. Thus, most clinicians recommend a minimum of six to eight months of adequate nonoperative treatment of synovitis before considering surgery.[3-6,8-10] If only one joint is the limiting factor one should probably try aspiration and steroid injection at least once before proceeding to synovectomy.

(2) Joint destruction is probably greater than shown on roentgenographs. Thus if cysts or erosive changes are already present there has been considerable articular damage, and secondary degenerative changes are certainly present. If synovectomy is to stop further articular damage, it must not be delayed beyond the point where significant architectural damage has already occurred.[3,4,8-10,13,14,18,19] Results are better when synovectomies are done before significant preoperative x-ray changes have occurred.

(3) As was proven in animal experiments as early as 1927, the synovial membrane will reform in a surprisingly short period.[20] A normal synovial membrane will reform in a month from residual hyperplastic synovium and fibroblastic metaplasia in situ. In one study in which adult patients were reevaluated by arthoscopy and biopsy after synovectomy, 95% had microscopic evidence of rheumatoid recurrence. However, most were still clinically better than before operation. Thus synovectomy is not curative but is a way of buying time for a joint until general remission occurs.

(4) Certain joints lend themselves readily to synovectomy, in particular the wrist, elbow, small joints of the hand, and especially the knee, the most commonly affected joints in JRA.[4,8-10,13,18] For technical reasons not more than 90% of the diseased synovium can be removed from these joints. Synovectomy is only occasionally useful for the hip partly because its involvement is less immediately noticeable, but also because exposure is technically more difficult, and because there is risk of aseptic necrosis of the femoral head.[6]

(5) In general a wet type of proliferative synovitis (boggy, with effusion) responds better to synovectomy than the so-called dry synovitis. The dry type is marked by minimal swelling and local

reaction, but progressive stiffness with little actual synovium found at time of surgery.[13,14]

(6) On the average properly chosen cooperative patients neither gain nor lose range of motion following synovectomy.[3,8-10,13] In order to avoid intraarticular and intramuscular fibrosis and subsequent loss of motion they must be able to perform range-of-motion exercises in the early postoperative period in the presence of pain. In fact, most orthopedists will routinely perform a manipulation under anesthesia two to three weeks after surgery if range of motion has not returned to its preoperative level. The necessity for a cooperative patient usually eliminates children under the age of seven or eight and those patients suffering from depression, who have been proven to recover least well from surgery.[21] This psychologic factor would also tend to eliminate patients with disseminated involvement of nearly every joint. One can do bilateral knee synovectomies simultaneously, but to operate on a patient who has every joint actively involved would be futile.[14]

(7) Relief of pain is the usual goal and will be achieved in the majority of patients although its absence is not necessarily a contraindication to synovectomy.[3,4,8-10,13] However, it is not always a significant problem and may be denied by nonambulatory physically inactive children.

(8) Despite the fact that synovectomy involves operating around epiphyses there is no evidence that it interferes with growth.[11] Thus it need not be delayed until skeletal maturity although the underlying disease frequently has already interfered with longitudinal growth.[22]

In summary, the ideal candidate for synovectomy would: (1) have pauciarticular disease of the knee or wrist; (2) be over eight years old without major psychological problems; (3) have a proliferative wet synovitis with continuous activity despite six to eight months of adequate medical treatment; and (4) have a fairly good range of motion with minimal x-ray changes. This is summarized in Table 1.

Table 1
Indications for Synovectomy

Relative Indications	Relative contraindications
Wet synovitis	Dry synovitis
Persistent disease activity over 6 to 8 months	Disease activity under 6 months
Patient over 8 years old	Patient under 7 years old
Cooperative patient	Psychological problems
Pauciarticular disease	Diffuse involvement
Lack of x-ray changes	Major joint destruction on x-ray
Significant pain and loss of function knee, wrist, elbow, hand	Intermetatarsal joints

BONE AND JOINT OPERATIONS

Arthrodesis

There are three important properties of a joint: range of motion, stability, and freedom from pain. Joint fusion sacrifices range of motion, but is generally an excellent way to relieve pain and instability in a particular joint. Its use in JRA is limited because successful function following fusion depends on the painless integrity of joints proximal and distal to the fused one. Also fusion is limited to extremities with involvement of only one joint, not a common situation in JRA. Instability alone is rarely an appropriate criterion since stiffness is more common. In fact, joints frequently fuse spontaneously in severe polyarticular disease, in which cases the goal is to allow fusion to occur in the best possible position for function (i.e., a right angle plantigrade foot).[18] In JRA the most useful places for surgical joint fusion are the wrist and finger interphalangeal joints and rarely, the cervical spine.

Osteotomy

Rotational or correctional osteotomies are generally reserved for older patients with fixed lateral angulatory or severe flexion deformities. Thus an ankle with 20° of motion between 40° and 60° of plantar flexion can have the range of motion changed to a more functional 20° about a neutral position. One of the disadvantages of osteotomy is that the limb must be immobilized until bony healing is complete, thereby producing stiffness in neighboring joints.[6]

Limb Length Equalization

This technique applies only to the lower extremities where asymmetric disease in the hips, knees, and ankles may lead to spontaneous growth discrepancies. When the leg length discrepancy is greater than one inch equalization can be performed in a growing child by arresting the growth of the longer side.[1,18] This is accomplished by inserting a bone graft across the epiphyseal plates of the knee on the longer leg (epiphysiodesis) or by inserting staples across the epiphyseal plate. When the short limb has caught up in length the staples can be removed and growth resumed, at least in theory. Usually growth arrest procedures are best delayed until the ages of 10 to 12 when careful planning using growth tables will allow prediction of how much relative arrest will occur at a specific skeletal age. Localized growth arrest is safer than leg lengthening, but not very appealing to a patient with generalized stunting which may be due to the disease itself. Luckily, most cases of leg length discrepancy in JRA are not great enough to require epiphysiodesis.

Epiphyseal stapling of one side of a joint has also been used for lateral deviation. Knee valgus has been treated by stapling of the medial side of the proximal tibia.[23]

Arthroplasty

Joint reconstruction is perhaps the most dramatic of the surgical procedures in JRA, however, other types of arthroplasty should not be forgotten. Excisional arthroplasty is an established technique, especially useful in the mature forefoot, elbow, and occasionally as a salvage procedure in the hip. By excising all joint surfaces, synovium, and capsule, the arthritic process is eliminated but joint stability and function are partially compromised depending on the anatomic situation. Interposition arthroplasty is accomplished by placing either autogenous fascia or an artificial substance between the joint surfaces after the diseased joint surfaces have been removed. Cup arthroplasty of the hip is the best known procedure of this type and has had considerable success in nonrheumatoid patients. In this procedure the femoral head and acetabulum are denuded of cartilage by reaming, and a metal cup is interposed. However, the failure rate of cup arthroplasty in JRA is high and it has been abandoned for this disease.[24] *Fascia lata* interposition of the elbow is a useful but seldom needed salvage procedure for the nearly ankylosed elbow.[4]

Total joint replacement is the most important recent advance in arthritis surgery. The earliest and most successful experience has been with hips, (Figure 1).[1,4,25,26] With available techniques relief of pain and attainment of a satisfactory range of motion are expected in most patients. Total knee replacement is also an established salvage procedure and early results are promising in the shoulder, elbow, wrist, and ankle. In these procedures the articular surfaces or entire bone ends are excised and replaced, usually with a metal component on one end and a carefully mated polyethylene component on the other joint surface. The parts are cemented in place with methyl methacrylate. It is preferable in most situations to use prostheses that are inherently unconstrained (not joined) and which depend on the normal musculoligamentous structures for stability. The periarticular soft tissue and muscle are then available to dampen the applied loads. Where these structures are inadequate constrained prosthesis with inherent stability such as a hinged knee must be used. Unfortunately, when using a constrained prosthesis the loads applied to one end are directly transmitted to the other end and magnified by the lever arm effect which results in loosening of the prosthesis and occasionally in metal fatigue and failure. In my opinion all constrained total joint replacements will eventually loosen. Besides this, joint implants have fractured, subluxed, eroded, become infected, and have induced fractures through the long bones at the end of the prosthetic implant. No prosthesis presently available, however, has actually worn down to the extent that it would have to be replaced. In fact no one really knows what to expect in terms of the life of cement or components even in unconstrained joints, since most long term clinical studies are in elderly and sedentary adults.

Early results are usually quite good. Since the only alternative may be a bed-chair existence, and since the activities of more severely affected patients are modest, surgeons are becoming more and more willing to implant total joints at earlier and earlier ages. The general prerequisite, however, is that skeletal maturity has been obtained (the epiphyseal plate is closed).

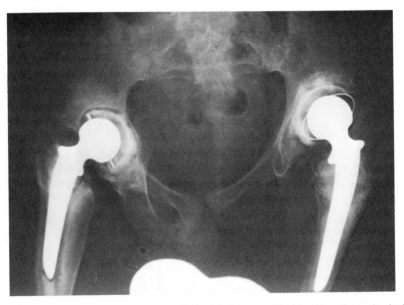

Figure 1. Radiograph of bilateral artificial hip joints in 19-year-old patient who had onset of disease at age 2. Bilateral cup arthroplasty operations at age 13 were unsuccessful because of persistent postoperative pain and stiffness. Total hip replacement at age 16 resulted in freedom from pain, good position, and ability to bear weight although stiffness persists.

236

A second major kind of implant arthroplasty is the flexible silastic type (Figure 2).[27] These are not cemented in place but simply positioned as spacers between two of the smaller bones after removal of the joint surfaces. Fixation is usually by intramedullary stems and they are most applicable to the small joints of the wrist and, especially, MP joints of the hand and great toe. A new joint capsule forms around these prostheses giving added stability. Results have generally been good in relieving pain and maintaining motion in young adult patients.

SPECIAL CONSIDERATIONS BEFORE PLANNING SURGICAL PROCEDURES

The decision to operate in JRA should usually be a combined decision by the orthopedist, rheumatologist, pediatrician, patient, and family. Certain common problems must always be weighed.

Stiffness

Postoperative immobilization should be the minimum possible and prolonged traction, spica casts, and bedrest should be avoided. A large

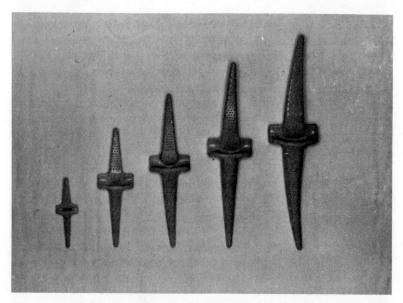

Figure 2. Flexible plastic implants to replace finger joints. The long stems fit the intramedullary canals of metacarpals and/or phalanges. Varied sizes that are available fit a wide range of sizes of bones.

operative hematoma is an invitation for postoperative fibrosis, therefore we recommend suction drainage and bulky compressive dressing with meticulous hemostasis.

Medications

Nearly all JRA patients are on aspirin. We have not found this to cause a problem with bleeding, although one should probably do preoperative coagulation studies. Some patients will be, or will have been, on steroids and will need to be covered for stress with added doses during operative and postoperative periods. These children will have a multitude of additional problems including skin fragility and delayed healing. They also tend to have increased osteoporosis making the risk of intraoperative fractures greater.

Psychology

Because of the disabling chronic nature of the disease many patients are depressed. A poor mental attitude is a relative contraindication to any elective surgical procedure. Of course, individualization is the key, but we have found it helpful to delay surgery if the patient can obtain preoperative counseling.

Growth Stunting

In the more severe cases growth is diffusely stunted. One should avoid procedures that would interfere with the limited growth available (i.e., total joint replacement in a skeletally immature patient). The bones are often so small that specifically designed, miniature prostheses are necessary.[25,26]

Anesthesia

Intubation may be difficult in JRA patients because of micrognathia, (Figure 3), temporomandibular or cricoarytenoid arthritis, or rigidity of the cervical spine, (Figure 4).[1,17] We have had to cancel cases on the operating table when anesthesiologists had not adequately recognized these problems beforehand. In patients with polyarticular disease, complete radiographic evaluation of the cervical spine is required

238

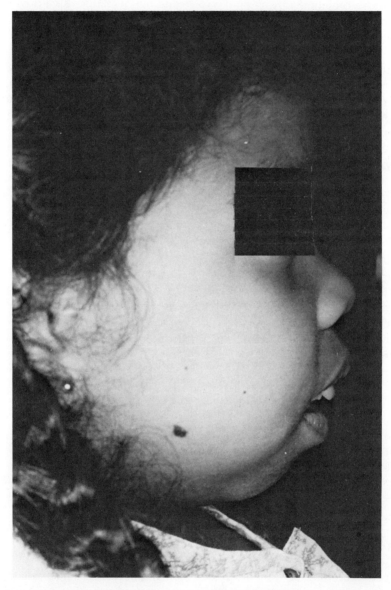

Figure 3. Girl with micrognathia. She also has fused cervical vertebrae. This combination of problems makes routine intubation for anesthesia difficult or impossible.

before planning anesthesia. An occasional difficulty is reduced chest compliance, probably due to costovertebral joint involvement. Regional anesthesia may be used, but requires a calm, cooperative and mature patient.

TREATMENT OF SPECIFIC AREAS

Spine

Involvement of the cervical spine is common and ankylosis at several zygapophyseal joints is a frequent outcome. Nearly always, however, a few levels remain mobile, (Figure 4). This situation allows some neck motion but places added stresses on the few remaining segments and can lead to localized instability with a potential for neurologic impairment.[28,29] The most common area of instability is the C1-C2 articulation, symptoms of which may be insidious and include occipital headache, lower extremity weakness, and tingling of the entire body with neck extension (Lhermitte's sign). A patient suspected of C1-C2 instability should have flexion and extension lateral x-rays of the cervical spine. Neurological sequelae are fortunately rare in JRA patients for two reasons: the upper canal is usually capacious enough to allow a significant degree of subluxation without cord impingement; and loose joints gradually regain a measure of stability. The rare children with neurological involvement should have posterior C1-C2 fusion with postoperative immobilization in a halo case.[4,28,29]

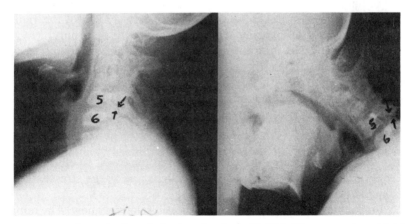

Figure 4. Radiograph of cervical spine of patient with JRA. The zygapophyseal joints are fused from C2 to C5, and only available flexion is at C5-C6. Normal extension is not possible.

prostheses will probably eventually break, however, fractured prostheses in the fingers are frequently asymptomatic and need not necessarily be replaced since a pseudocapsular fibrous tissue forms around the prosthesis and affords significant stability. If subluxation does result after failure of the prostheses they can be easily replaced.

Hips

Until recently the hip has not been the site of much surgical treatment in JRA. Since it is so deeply situated anatomically, it is much less accessible for clinical evaluation of synovitis, joint deformity, or local treatment by injection. Additionally, the most common deformity, flexion contracture, is compensated for by the patient by increasing lumbar lordosis. Finally, the hip is rarely the first or only joint involved. Thus early hip involvement may go unnoticed by the clinician and the child may not complain of hip symptoms until there is advanced destruction.[6,18]

Synovectomy of the hip has been recommended but is not often performed. It is a much more extensive procedure and must often be combined with capsulotomy and muscle release to correct the flexion and adduction contractures. To remove most of the synovium adequately would require dislocation of the femoral head and this has the theoretical risk of inducing aseptic necrosis.[6,8,9] Thus although it may occasionally be indicated, synovectomy is difficult to perform well. Soft tissue releases about the hip also have a marked tendency to postoperative stiffness. In some patients heterotopic bone may form thus eliminating gains made at the time of surgery. We have not performed any synovectomies of the hip.

Hip fusion should probably not be considered in JRA patients since its success depends on normal knee and spine mechanics, a situation rarely present in JRA.

Total hip replacement is the procedure of choice for the young adult patient with sequelae of JRA since relief of pain and gain in motion are relatively predictable and series of patients are being reported with increasingly lower age limits.[1,4,26] It should never be done in a growing child, but epiphyseal plates are often closed early by the disease. Particularly small components may be needed because of the small bone size, and these must be compared to preoperative x-rays to make sure that they will fit, (Figure 5). Inadequate bone stock is a contraindication to total hip replacement. Children will have all of the usual problems that adults have with joint replacement including loosening, infection (1% to 2%), metal failure, etc. The major dif-

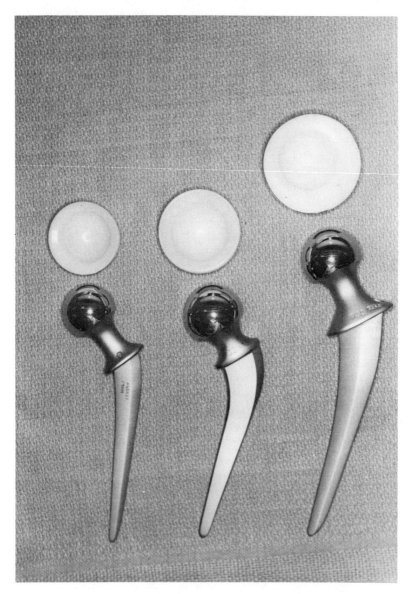

Figure 5. Varied sizes of total hip replacement components. Careful matching of size of component to size of child's bone is essential before starting surgery for total hip replacement.

ference is that children will have many more years in which to have these complications. Undoubtedly with time many if not all the total hips implanted now in youngsters will need revision, thus it is not an operation to be undertaken lightly. Nevertheless, if it is the only way to allow someone out of a wheelchair it should not be withheld. It is hoped that future mechanical and design improvements will lessen the chance of complication.

Knees

The knee is the most commonly affected joint in JRA and in many ways causes the most disability.[13,17] It is the most important joint in the lower extremity for gait and has the least amount of compensatory mechanism for loss of function. For a weight-bearing joint it is poorly designed, having no intrinsic bony stability and being totally dependent on ligament and muscular integrity. Extension of the knee (as for example, in a long leg brace) tremendously increases the work of walking by lengthening the lever arm of the leg. A fixed flexion contracture is even more devastating since the muscle effort required to walk increases by 6% for each degree of flexion deformity.[30] To prevent buckling when standing on a 40° fixed flexion contracture, the quadriceps must exert a force of over 240% of body weight. Any loss of knee motion makes walking immediately more fatiguing especially in the chronically ill child. However, the joint is superficial, deformity is readily measured, and it is easily accessible to surgery and is probably the ideal joint for early synovectomy.[4,18] If appropriate criteria are met (Table 1) most published reports claim good results, especially in relief of pain.[3,8,9,13] Knee synovectomy can be performed through a median parapatellar incision or through a shorter medial and lateral incision. I prefer the former. It must allow enough exposure to remove at least 80% to 90% of the diseased synovium. It is important to save the loose areolar fat in the suprapatellar area to prevent adhesions of the quadriceps which would limit flexion. The knee should be immobilized in maximal extension postoperatively and range-of-motion exercises started in seven to 10 days. Manipulation of the knee under anesthesia is necessary if range of motion is slow in returning.

The most common knee deformity is flexion contracture, often associated with a valgus deformity. When contracture is greater than 20°, unresponsive to bracing, and the patient is a walker or potential walker, a posterior capsular release is indicated. Most clinicians describe lengthening of both medial and lateral hamstrings with capsulotomy, however, since the knees are in valgus, lateral structures are relatively shorter. I therefore do not usually lengthen the medial hamstrings. A complete posterior capsulotomy is necessary if any correction is to be obtained. Because there is a marked tendency for posterior subluxation of the tibia when previously contracted knees are straightened, one should always obtain radiographs of the knees postoperatively. I prefer to use parallel posterior medial and lateral incisions with the patient in prone position which allows excellent visualization of the entire posterior capsule. I usually divide the anterior cruciate ligament which is a major factor in posterior subluxation.[18] The neurovascular structures, especially the peroneal nerve, must be isolated and protected during the surgical procedure and are usually limiting factors in the amount of correction obtainable. If full correction cannot be obtained at surgery, one may use postoperative, serial, wedging casts. The following are important: (1) The cast should be well padded over the knee and posterior calf area, (2) I believe a pin should be used through the tibia so that the forces will be applied directly to bone, and (3) the rate of extension of the joint should not exceed the ability of the neurovascular bundle to adapt to the stretching of its tissues. Additionally, wedges should not be made at the anatomic area of the knee joint. Rather, wedging should be performed approximately three to five inches above the knee so that the tibia is brought forward in addition to being extended. Range-of-motion exercises should be begun within two to three weeks after soft tissue release but the knee must be protected in extension in an orthosis for at least three to six months. If the flexion deformity of the knee is even greater (over 60°) an extension osteotomy of the distal femur will transfer the arc of motion to a more useful range.[4] Also severe valgus deformity can be corrected by osteotomy if the joint surfaces are relatively preserved. If joint surfaces are totally destroyed one might as well wait and perform a total knee replacement near skeletal maturity.

Total knee replacement is rapidly becoming the procedure of choice for the young adult patient with severe sequelae from JRA. However, the "state of art" is not as satisfactory as with total hip replacement. There are myriad different knee designs available which makes it difficult to choose any one type and improvements are constantly being made in design and material. None have been tested for long times in younger patients. The two general classifications are hinged (constrained) and surface replacement (unconstrained). The hinge prostheses give immediate results which are usually excellent but probably will all eventually loosen or break and should be reserved for marginal walkers or for patients with no ligamentous support, i.e., those who have had a previous spontaneous ankylosis.[4] One should attempt to use a surface replacement type of knee replacement.

Foot and Ankle

Involvement of the ankle, tarsal, and metatarsal joints is usual in patients with persistent disease in whom there is a strong tendency for spontaneous ankylosis. Every attempt should be made to insure that the foot is maintained in a plantigrade position. Synovitis is often insidious and synovectomy is rarely done, although possible. Arthrodesis of the ankle is quite functional, however, when joint involvement is severe enough to indicate ankle arthrodesis, simply waiting and bracing will probably result in a spontaneous ankylosis. If a severe contracture occurs in the hindfoot (usually equinus), tendoachilles lengthening and posterior capsulotomy of the ankle may be indicated although in practice this is rarely done. Instead we have used supramalleolar osteotomy to obtain a plantigrade foot. In this procedure a wedge of bone based anteriorly is taken from the distal tibia just above the malleoli and the foot brought up, (Figure 6). With severe valgus or varus of the heel an appropriate osteotomy of the heel can be used to correct the foot to the midposition if shoe modification and inserts are not adequate.

JRA patients may have a variety of problems in the forefoot including bunions, metatarsalgia, metatarsophalangeal dislocations, and hammer toes. In young adults with these problems excisional arthroplasty of the MP joints is usually an excellent procedure.[31] It is occasionally necessary to fuse or excise interphalangeal joints of toes

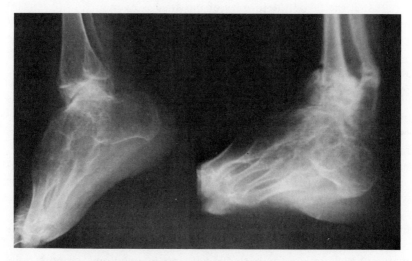

Figure 6. Radiograph of ankle before and after wedge osteotomies of tibia and fibula to allow dorsiflexion of foot into a plantigrade position after spontaneous fusion of ankle. Position allows comfortable walking gait.

to correct severe clawing which is permissible before skeletal maturity.

CONCLUSIONS

The multiple surgical procedures useful in treatment of JRA are not radical alternatives to failure of other forms of treatment. Nor is surgery curative, but it is another mode of control. Synovectomy can temporarily relieve pain and buy time. Osteotomy, contracture release, and fusion can correct deformity and improve function. Total joint replacement can relieve pain and restore motion, but long-term results are unknown and many improvements will have to be made. Special precautions are needed in planning any of the surgical procedures in JRA patients because of cervical spine involvement, difficulty with intubation, growth stunting, poor bony stock, and often significant psychologic problems.

REFERENCES

1. Arden, G.P. Surgical treatment of Still's disease. *Ann R Coll Surg Engl.* 53:288–99, 1973.
2. Jakubowski, S., and Ruszczynska, J. The possibility of surgical treatment in cases of juvenile rheumatoid arthritis. *Acta Rheum Scand.* 13:113–18, 1967.
3. Kampner, S.L., and Ferguson, A.B. Efficacy of synovectomy in juvenile rheumatoid arthritis. *Clin Orthop.* 88:94–109, 1972.
4. Murray, W.R. Juvenile rheumatoid arthritis. *Curr Pract Orthop Surg.* 6:171–212, 1975.
5. Barry, P.E., and Stillman, J.S. Characteristics of juvenile rheumatoid arthritis: its medical and orthopaedic management. *Orthop Clin North Am.* 6:641–53, 1975.
6. Albright, J.A., Albright, J.P., and Ogden, J.A. Synovectomy of the hip in juvenile rheumatoid arthritis. *Clin Orthop.* 106:48–55, 1975.
7. Anderson, L.D., and Heppenstall, M. Synovectomy of the elbow and excision of the radial head in rheumatoid arthritis. Edited by R.L. Cruess and N.S. Mitchell. In *Surgery of Rheumatoid Arthritis.* Philadelphia: J.B. Lippincott, 1971.
8. Eyring, E.J. The therapeutic potential of synovectomy in juvenile rheumatoid arthritis. *Arthritis Rheum.* 11:688–92, 1968.
9. Eyring, E.J., Longert, A., and Bass, J.C. Synovectomy in juvenile rheumatoid arthritis. *J Bone Joint Surg.* 53A:638–51, 1971.
10. Fink, C.W., Baum, J., Paradies, L.H., and Carrell, B.C. Synovectomy in juvenile rheumatoid arthritis. *Ann Rheum Dis.* 28:612–16, 1969.
11. Garrett, A.L., and Campbell, C. Synovectomy in children. Edited by R.L. Cruess and N.S. Mitchell. In *Surgery of Rheumatoid Arthritis.* Philadelphia: J.B. Lippincott, 1971.

248

12. Goel, K.M., and Shanks, R.A. Follow-up study of 100 cases of juvenile rheumatoid arthritis. *Ann Rheum Dis.* 33:25–31, 1974.

13. Granberry, W.M., and Brewer, E.J. Results of synovectomy in children with rheumatoid arthritis. *Clin Orthop.* 101:120–6, 1974.

14. Isaacson, A.S. Operative procedures on patients with juvenile rheumatoid arthritis. American Academy of Orthopedic Surgeons, *Instructional Course Lectures 23*, 1974, p. 37–40.

15. London, P.S. Synovectomy of the knee in rheumatoid arthritis. *J Bone Joint Surg.* 37B:392–9, 1955.

16. Swett, P.O. Synovectomy in chronic infectious arthritis. *J Bone Joint Surg.* 6:800, 1924.

17. Laaksonen, A.-L. A prognostic study of juvenile rheumatoid arthritis: analysis of 544 cases. *Acta Rheum Scand.* 166 (suppl):16–80, 1966.

18. Granberry, W.M., and Brewer, E.J. Orthopaedic management of juvenile rheumatoid arthritis. Edited by E.J. Brewer. In *Juvenile Rheumatoid Arthritis.* Philadelphia: W.B. Saunders, 1971.

19. Mongan, E.S., Boger, W.M., Gilliland, B.C., and Meyerowitz, S. Synovectomy in rheumatoid arthritis. *Arthritis Rheum.* 13:761–8, 1970.

20. Wolcott, W.E. Regeneration of the synovial membrane following typical synovectomy. *J Bone Joint Surg.* 9:67–78, 1927.

21. Patzakis, M.J., Mills, D.M., Bartholomew, B.A. et al. A visual histological and enzymatic study of regenerating rheumatoid synovium in the synovectomized knee. *J Bone Joint Surg.* 55A:287–300, 1973.

22. Marmour, L. *Surgery of Rheumatoid Arthritis.* Philadelphia: Lea and Febiger, 1967, p. 252.

23. Ansell, B.M., Arden, G.P., and McLennan, I. Valgus knee deformities in children with chronic polyarthritis treated by epiphyseal stapling. *Arch Dis Child.* 45:388–92, 1970.

24. Lang, A.G., and Klassen, R.A. Cup arthroplasties in teenagers and children. *J Bone Joint Surg.* 59A:444–50, 1977.

25. Arden, G.P., Ansell, B.M., and Hunter, M.J. Total hip replacement in juvenile chronic polyarthritis and ankylosing spondylitis. *Clin Orthop.* 84:130–6, 1972.

26. Bisla, R.J., Inglis, A.E., and Ranawat, C.S. Joint replacement surgery in patients under thirty. *J Bone Joint Surg.* 58A:1098–1103, 1976.

27. Swanson, A.B. Flexible implant arthroplasty for arthritic finger joints. *J Bone Joint Surg.* 54A:435–55, 1972.

28. Ferlic, D.C., Clayton, M.L., Leidholt, J.D., and Gamble, W.E. Surgical treatment of the symptomatic unstable cervical spine in rheumatoid arthritis. *J Bone Joint Surg.* 57A:349–54, 1975.

29. Thomas, W.H. Surgical management of the rheumatoid cervical spine. *Orthop Clin North Am.* 6:793–800, 1975.

30. Perry, J., Antonelli, D., and Ford, W. Analysis of knee joint forces during flexed-knee stance. *J Bone Joint Surg.* 57A:961–7, 1975.

31. Clayton, M.L. Surgery of the forefoot in rheumatoid arthritis. *Clin Orthop.* 16:136–40, 1960.

17 Psychodynamics of Juvenile Rheumatoid Arthritis

Bernhard H. Singsen
Mark A. Johnson
Bram A. Bernstein

The concept of the team approach to health care for children with chronic disease is widely accepted. In practice, unfortunately, it is still evident that far too little attention is paid to the psychosocial aspects of chronic illnesses. In this chapter we will examine the literature regarding psychosocial consequences of chronic disease in childhood, explore psychosocial factors in adult rheumatoid arthritis (RA), review the few investigations of psychodynamics of juvenile rheumatoid arthritis (JRA) and, finally, present a clinician's (nonpsychiatrist's) scheme of approach to and management of the emotional consequences of JRA.

As implied above, almost any discussion of psychosocial aspects of a chronic disease such as JRA has an inherent bias. A review of the large body of literature about the interrelationship between arthritis and personality reveals a recurring suggestion that patients with RA have common psychosocial characteristics, and that from these one may propose the existence of a "rheumatoid personality." We will demonstrate that there is no conclusive answer as to whether the majority of patients with RA exhibit specific premorbid psychosocial or personality characteristics. Rather, our bias is that current evidence and our experience show that the most commonly observed personality characteristics are results of the consequences of the disease process.

AN OVERVIEW OF CHRONIC DISEASE IN CHILDHOOD

There is an extensive literature regarding the psychologic and social consequences of chronic disease in childhood.[1-9] Most of these reports do not deal directly with JRA, but many aspects of their approach are readily applicable to and can be easily integrated with this disease.

Maddison and Raphael pointed out that evaluations of the psychologic and social consequences of chronic illness can produce very different findings depending on the depth of the study.[1] As an example, Brazelton, et al. found that many of the really relevant anxieties and concerns of children with rheumatic fever and of their mothers, did not become evident until after 10 to 15 detailed one-hour interviews.[2] With this background it is easier to understand why physicians with their comprehensive responsibilities are likely to accept good behavior or passive conformity among patients as evidence that things are going well and that no psychologic consequences of note need be anticipated.[1]

Chronic disease in childhood has the potential to affect greatly the psychosocial development of the child. Specific developmental crises may be inadequately resolved depending on their nature, age of the child, and form of chronic illness.[1,3,4] If, for example, onset of arthritis is between one to three years, there may be an intensification of maternal control, limitation of the child's opportunity for self-expression, and increased evidence of passivity and a sense of helplessness, all of which may interfere with achieving autonomy. The development of conscience is believed to be maximal between ages four and five, when onset of chronic illness may lead to marked feelings of guilt and loss of initiative if the child believes that disease is "punishment" for forbidden thoughts or feelings. Between ages six and 11, chronic disease may lead to feelings of inadequacy or inferiority. Finally, the development or continuation of a chronic disease such as JRA in adolescence may result in limited ability to develop adequate concepts of role and identity.

In their study of family adaptation to the child with cystic fibrosis McCollum and Gibson describe four stages of adjustment to chronic or fatal illness: prediagnostic, confrontational, long-term, and terminal.[8] These concepts are applicable to JRA.

In the prediagnostic state parental concern is aroused and medical advice is repeatedly sought. Incomplete or incorrect diagnoses, parental overconcern, and the physician's failure to ameliorate symptoms, often prolong this stage and lead to parental mistrust of and hostility toward the medical profession. This stage is also crucial because of its significant effects on the child-parent relationship when parental feelings of self-doubt or reproach may lead to despair, frank hostility towards the child, or guilt.

The confrontational stage is that period of acute stress associated with confirmation of the diagnosis. This period is of variable duration and described as one of intense anxiety and acute anticipatory mourning reaction because of the potentially fatal illness. This stage has clear parallels with systemic sclerosis or lupus erythematosus, but probably differs only in degree for any chronic illness which may limit the child's potential and the parents' aspirations for the child. At this time parental defense mechanisms are mobilized and may include transient detachment or absence of affect, feelings of disbelief, and denial. Physician counselling and educational efforts are rapidly forgotten and random attempts to gather positive information from a variety of nonprofessional sources frequently follow. Anger directed against previous physicians who failed to make the correct diagnosis was found to be common. At times anger was also directed against the marital partner for his/her supposed genetic contributions or lack of concern, or against the religious faith that had failed to protect their child. Anxiety was further heightened by feelings of helplessness in altering the disease outcome and the adequacy of the basic parental function of protectiveness was thus threatened.

Major issues at this time also included: Where to live relative to specialty clinical centers? How to absorb the potentially catastrophic costs of specialized care? How to master all the therapeutic techniques that need be provided at home? Many of these observations regarding the cystic child and his family are clearly applicable to the child newly diagnosed as having JRA.

The challenge for many parents in the third stage of long-term adaptation is to maintain a relationship with an afflicted child which can afford some parental gratification and yet fulfill the child's physical and psychologic needs. The illness affects family routines and stimulates awareness of the child's prognosis. Critical issues involving requirements for medical or physical therapy serve as foci for parental concern and impinge upon childhood development. Major developmental requirements for children of varying ages are therefore impeded and frustrated.

At this point it is relevant to consider pain as a factor in childhood chronic disease. In most chronic conditions it is not a major factor; it may result from diagnostic tests, or occur during exacerbations of some diseases, but rarely, except in JRA, is it an ever-present concomitant of disease. Younger children can distinguish only rarely between pain associated with an illness and that caused by treatment.[1] In addition patients of any age may associate pain with concepts of punishment or persecution. Rage or a desire for revenge are common consequences in both parent and patient, which may foster dependency and regression on the part of the child. Care of the painful chronically ill child will provide some increased gratification of his dependency needs, but parental feelings of worthlessness and helplessness may result if the pain is not relieved.

Alternatively, excessive gratification of dependency needs may retard maturation and fixate the child at a stage in which passively received parental attention provides maximum pleasure. This may create conflict for the child who previously had taken pride in performance of certain activities, and whose acceptance of responsibilities can now no longer be undertaken. The same conflict will also appear in the child who sees peers or siblings attain new levels which he or she cannot achieve. Maddison and Raphael point out that regression or a return to more infantile behavior may be particularly marked in the patient for whom achievement of independence has always been a struggle.[1] In children who are stressed by their disease or by conflict regarding their dependency needs regression may make disease management significantly more difficult, and occasionally may lead to psychologic defects which persist beyond disease remission.

Physical limitations in activity may also be of consequence for the developing child because intellectual development partly depends upon interaction with an adequately stimulating environment. Restriction of play removes an important channel for the resolution of conflict, particularly if adequate alternatives are not provided by sensitive parents or other members of a therapeutic team. Some believe that restriction of activity will inevitably cause an increase in a child's fantasy life as an alternate way to control tensions and it is suggested that the child who complains about and resists restrictions is probably dealing with limitations in a healthier fashion than the child who exhibits "good behavior" or "adjustment."[1] The patient who makes the work of the health team easier may well be demonstrating apathy, withdrawal, or early psychologic crippling.

RHEUMATOID ARTHRITIS—
PSYCHOSOCIAL CONCEPTS

The Adult Literature

Interest in the interaction of psyche and soma in patients with RA has existed at least since 1939 when Cobb and associates concluded that emotional stress was a precipitating environmental factor in the etiology of RA.[10] More recently, King[11] and Wolff[12] have critically reviewed the status of psychosocial contributions to the disease. King reviewed 50 earlier reports, but noted that only two studies had included controls and that most studies were descriptive, used poor diagnostic criteria, and did not include longitudinal assessment.[11]

Wolff raised four questions with which the present authors concur as a sensible approach to reviewing the literature and as a framework for developing future studies: "(1) Is it indeed correct that the majority of RA patients evidence some common and typical personality and psychosocial characteristics? (2) If, indeed, there exist common or typical personality and psychosocial characteristics are they specific to RA? (3) If it can be demonstrated that there are indeed certain personality and psychosocial characteristics specific to RA are these premorbid personality traits and psychosocial constellations or are they secondary to the physical disease? (4) If there are personality and psychosocial characteristics specific to RA what is the mechanism whereby these behavioral factors precipitate or influence the physical disease?"[12]

Attempts to answer these questions have met with varying degrees of success. An index of rheumatoid arthritis, designed by King and Cobb, has been employed in several studies to show that RA patients demonstrate "contained hostility."[13-15] These investigators also observed that men with rheumatoid disease had little education, low income, and were more frequently divorced.[16] Women with RA generally had less education, "worried" more than controls, had four or more children, had much covert hostility and low overt aggressiveness, had increased conflict about controlling anger associated with feelings of guilt, and had large social class differences in the marriage patterns of their parents and themselves.

Scotch and Geiger,[17] and Moos,[18] have concluded that these and other psychosocial studies frequently lack scientific precision. They note the absence of important information about patient characteristics, lack of heterogeneity within patient populations, inadequate statements about how many psychosocial variables were examined in comparison to those believed to be significant, lack of adequate controls and, perhaps most importantly, a lack of knowledge about the relationship between statements made by the RA patient and his or her actual behavior. Moos[12] nevertheless concurred with previous studies which showed that emotional factors have a definite role in RA. But, as suggested by Wolff,[12,19] many studies do not furnish enough valid information to document whether similar emotional factors are found in other disabling conditions, or if they are specific to RA. Wolff further noted the difficulty in finding a disease comparable to RA in terms of pain, progressive crippling, and alternating exacerbations and remissions for use as a control condition. This difficulty is demonstrated by one study which used ulcer patients as "controls."[20]

In general, two problems are apparent about psychologic investigations of patients with RA. The first is that the majority of studies are retrospective and rely heavily on projective testing and interviews, both of which tend to limit objectivity. The second observation is that even the more quantifiable and objective tests, such as the Minnesota Multiphasic Personality Inventory (MMPI) and Cattell's 16 Personality Factors Questionnaire (16 PF), are rarely applied prospectively from disease onset. Two exceptions are noteworthy for their prospective approach and those studies were largely limited to the relationship between pain and mood as they affected outcome in a rehabilitation setting.[21,22] Moldofsky and Chester found a significant correlation between pain, whether measured subjectively or objectively, and mood patterns in RA.[21] They observed a "synchronous" group in whom anxiety decreased as pain abated and a "paradoxical" group in whom anxiety or hopelessness increased as pain lessened. Their follow-up of these groups showed an improved outcome for the "synchronous" group, suggesting that patterns of pain and mood might have predictive value. Wolff also observed that tolerance to pain influenced the rehabilitation of arthritic patients.[22]

Finally, Meyerowitz[23] discussed the grouping of psychosocial factors in RA into three categories which are not dissimilar to those suggested by Wolff. They are (1) a specificity hypothesis wherein patients developing RA are characterized by definite psychologic traits presumed to have existed prior to disease onset, (2) a disease-onset hypothesis wherein there is an association between psychologic states, certain life experiences, and the onset of RA, and (3) a disease-course hypothesis wherein identifiable psychologic responses in RA patients influence the course of disease.

The Pediatric Literature

Investigations of the psychosocial dynamics of JRA have only recently begun to appear. They are few in number and generally do not achieve the sophistication of literature regarding adults.

In 1954 Blom and Nicholls published the first observations of emotional factors in patients with JRA.[24] Unfortunately this report is almost entirely anecdotal although many of the concepts discussed are valid for any poorly understood chronic disease. These include: (1) significance of onset of arthritis during critical phases in the emotional development of the child, (2) recurrence or aggravation of arthritis in relation to an emotionally charged situation, (3) an unusual degree of fantasy explanations about arthritis (by both parents and children), and (4) severe separation reactions including depression, feelings of abandonment, and desertion at the time of hospitalizations. These authors observed extreme mother-child interdependency, marked mood disturbances in the children and inability of the children to express their feelings. Ambivalence, conflict, sadistic fantasies, and feeding difficulties were found. The effects of pain, chronicity of disease, and perceptions of the child's future were not discussed. These authors concluded that it is difficult to state how emotional factors are related to onset of arthritis but that recurrences and speed of recovery in JRA are influenced by emotional factors. Their most significant observation was that children with JRA often had an infantile personality structure growing out of a long sustained conflict situation in which the outstanding element was inability of the child to achieve separateness from the mother. This study is also instructive because it is one of the few with longitudinal assessment of the children.

Cleveland, Reitman, and Brewer[25] studied the interplay of psychologic factors and chronic somatic illness in JRA using a battery of tests of children, standard one-hour interviews with the mothers, and a comparison with similar data collected from children with chronic asthma. These authors stressed their belief that arthritic children are "unusually expressive in physical and muscle action" and suggest, and we agree, that it is important to design a therapeutic regimen with maximum permissible physical activity, pointing out that any degree of sensory deprivation may be detrimental.

The major difficulty with the hypothesis regarding premorbid physical activity as suggested by Wolff, is that data derived from retrospective questioning about activity are probably invalid.[12] It is a natural response derived from anxiety and grief, for parents to remember their now limited child as previously very active while present limitations increase.

Cleveland, et al. also noted the frequency of guilt and depression in mothers of JRA patients, but stressed their lack of clear understanding of the effects of this on the children.[25] Controls in this study were asthmatic children who were tested by a different psychologist, and who were comparable only by virtue of similar chronicity of their illness. The important concern continues to be that there may be no disease with pain, chronicity, immobilization, and exacerbations and remissions which allows for significant psychologic comparison with RA or JRA.

Cleveland and Brewer later wrote a more general review of their experience and opinion discussing the reactions of child and parent to JRA as a disease, and to the therapeutic program.[26] They reviewed theories about relationships between psyche and soma and described difficulties of performing psychologic research in arthritis. However, no pragmatic plan of approach to arthritic children and their parents was offered. Indeed, we have found that concrete suggestions about dealing with the psychosocial consequences of arthritis are almost never made in the current literature.

Meyerowitz, et al. investigated eight monozygotic twin sets discordant for RA, three pairs of whom were under 18 years old when studied.[27] Clinical, genetic, and particularly, psychologic aspects were studied in detail. The authors observed a conspicuous preference for active lives in both members of the twin sets, defining activity in broad dimensions of mobility in sports, traveling, moving to different homes, and a characteristic style of managing, assuming responsibility, and helping and taking care of others. These investigators found "entrapment" to be the most striking psychosocial finding in the affected twin. This term denotes stress on an individual who feels compelled to meet the demands of a close individual, object, or situation. The response to this demand is heightened activity in the broad sense of the word, but the entrapment eventually limits the patient. The increased activity was inferred by Meyerowitz and his colleagues to be derived from a specific style of ego functioning but not a defensive reaction. They observed no consistent relationship between personality characteristics and the occurrence of RA.

This study is important for several reasons. It defines activity more broadly as a manifestation of ego functioning and therefore devalues the concept of increased activity having a direct effect on the musculoskeletal system. It also points out that different personality characteristics play a role in determining which life events are psychologically stressful for each RA patient. This appears reasonable to us because stress thus becomes one of multiple unknown pathogenetic factors in RA without the implication that personality characteristics are directly related to disease occurrence.

Up to the present time (1978), many reports regarding the psycho-social events surrounding JRA have come from psychologists or psychiatrists at centers where large numbers of patients are available for study. Strangely, the well-known pediatric and adult rheumatologists presumably involved in the medical care of these children are not usually coauthors, or listed in acknowledgments. We believe this has led to a number of problems: (1) medical facts are omitted or distorted through lack of medical experience or intimate knowledge of the literature, (2) medical reports are cited to uphold a particular psychologic point of view, although subsequent research has invalidated the data cited, (3) medical reports which support an author's point of view are cited and there is little discussion of others which may negate it.

A case in point is a study by Heisel of stress as an etiologic factor in JRA.[28] The premise of the article, life-changes as etiologic factors in JRA, is based on a retrospective chart review to establish date of disease onset. It is well known by pediatric rheumatologists that a specific date of onset of JRA may be very difficult to define. Meticulous history-taking will often reveal a long period of insidious, slowly progressive symptoms which finally culminate in overt disease, these symptoms frequently having occurred over months or years prior to an established diagnosis. Heisel assumes that JRA is a psychosomatic disease and concludes that it has "specific trigger" events.

We are in strong disagreement with the concept that one can employ an operative pre-study definition of JRA as a psychosomatic disease, particularly if there are no data beyond the obvious emotional problems which beset children with JRA to support this point of view. Given the nature of the disease, one must be careful in evaluating the validity of data linking it with lifestyle, although it is tempting to relate emotionally charged events to the onset of a disease of which etiology is unknown, and where emotional difficulties are manifest.

It is obvious that emotional factors *are* related to the manner in which patients cope with the severity and chronicity of JRA. It is certainly a common anecdotal observation that many children handle their disease better when emotionally charged situations are defused. Whether the charging and defusing of crises can be related to disease onset and remission, respectively, remains an unanswered question but what can be concluded is that prospective, more detailed, meticulously organized, cooperative studies involving a comprehensive health-care team are required to provide answers about the interrelationships between psyche and soma at the onset of JRA.

Rimon and coworkers reported studies of 54 patients with JRA.[30] Their findings are based on interviews with patients and relatives, a "symptom profile" completed by various medical personnel, and a rating scale of personality, behavior, and psychiatric symptoms. The rating scale and its relative weighting of variables is not described. Much of this investigation is anecdotal in nature and appears designed to agree or disagree with the previous literature rather than to develop and analyze independent information. The study is not longitudinal, never addresses the concept of controls, and also appears biased by emphasis on the importance of psychologically charged events antecedent to developing JRA. The authors conclude that two main categories of patients with JRA exist: (1) those with a hereditary predisposition to JRA and whose disease is little influenced by environmental change, and (2) those in whom onset and progression of disease are associated with emotionally charged events. The complex literature regarding definition of hereditary predisposition is never discussed. There is no discussion as to whether the defined life stress factors are more common in the study group than in other age and socioeconomically adjusted control populations. Perhaps the most important point made by these investigators is that "more systematic psychotherapeutic methods and social counselling are needed, especially at the onset of illness, and . . . there is a definite need for a 'psychodynamic diagnosis' of the entire family."[30]

In our view the best investigation about psychologic aspects of JRA is that of McAnarney and her colleagues.[31] Their approach, which is also our own bias, is stated in the introduction: "The effect of physical disease on the developing child's emotional and social health is as important an area for investigation as are efforts to establish a causative relationship of psychological factors to the etiology of presumed psychosomatic disorders."[31] Matched by age and socioeconomics this study used controls and relatively precise techniques for gathering and analyzing data. Several important findings were made. Emotional health was judged to be excellent in only 36% of JRA patients, versus 60% of controls and 30% of the arthritic children had low adjustment ratings compared to 9% of controls. Contrary to what might be expected those arthritic children with minimal or no disability had significantly more psychosocial problems than their more disabled peers. These differences were not eliminated when duration of illness, degree of family disruption, and amount of time the mother spent in school was analyzed. It appeared that the parents of the nondisabled

arthritics had a poorer understanding of the disease, felt it was hereditary, and failed to acknowledge that JRA had any impact on their child's
behavior, schooling, social relations, or outlook for the future. The
authors' discussion of psychosocial impact on the relatively nondisabled child is important. They suggest that teachers and
"significant others" may make fewer allowances for these patients
with invisible disease than for the most obviously handicapped child
who receives generous allowances for his inability to keep up with
social, scholastic, and developmental expectations.

The implications of the study by McAnarney et al.[31] with which
we totally concur, are that provision for adequate psychosocial support
for arthritic children and their families must be an integral part of outpatient services, and that special efforts will be required for both the
disabled and nondisabled groups to break defenses and ensure that
anxieties, conflicts, and concerns about the future are identified early.
They emphasize that frequent contact with the school regarding performance and behavior is vital, and stress the importance of a program
which reevaluates the arthritic child psychologically at regular intervals with the same intensity as physicians do medically.

Henoch and her colleagues surveyed 88 children with JRA in an
attempt to find characteristics which might have etiologic significance.[32] The most striking finding was an almost three times
greater incidence of parental divorce, separation, death, or adoption of
the afflicted child in the JRA population than in the population of the
urban county served by the group doing the study (Monroe County,
New York). However, in only 48% of 31 affected children had these
events taken place within approximately two years of disease onset.
This spread of timing between onset of physical disease and of presumed significant psychological stress is not discussed. N.E. Penn and
S. Emerson looked at JRA from a different point of view (personal
communication). Twenty-four women with onset of arthritis before 16
years of age were identified as young adults (mean age 25.8 years) and
tested by several psychologic instruments, principally the MMPI. This
approach might be faulted for the small patient sample and lack of
controls, but yielded several important conclusions. All patients demonstrated some difficulty with masculinity-femininity differentiation.
Also, the later the age of disease onset and the longer the duration of
active painful JRA, the more anxiety, social shyness, and ego instability developed suggesting that particularly close attention should be
directed towards the psychosocial adjustment of preadolescents and
teenagers who develop the disease.

At this time it is relevant to restate our bias that many of the
currently available studies of these aspects of JRA are at least partially

anecdotal, nonlongitudinal, poorly controlled, inherently biased in viewpoint, and pay inadequate attention to the multiplicity of variables. In our opinion it is noteworthy that no such study has come from the collaboration of a psychiatrist or psychologist with a strong background in chronic childhood disease, particularly JRA, and a pediatric rheumatologist with intimate knowledge of the disease's medical and emotional aspects. A broadly applicable study of these problems will require (1) a major funding source, (2) a longitudinal perspective which begins evaluation as close to the start of the disease as possible, (3) as wide a range of testing and statistical methods as possible, (4) carefully selected controls, and (5) a lack of bias regarding points to be proven.

AN APPROACH TO MANAGEMENT

Perhaps most distressing about the current literature is the almost complete lack of attention given to management of common emotional difficulties that JRA patients and their families encounter. Recognition of them, and awareness of their likelihood is central to adequate treatment. We have been impressed with the universality of these difficulties, the frequency with which they remain unstated, and the persistence which may be required to bring them to a conscious verbal level where they can be explored. There is undoubtedly no right way to deal with them but awareness, sensitivity, and patience are the major prerequisites for effectiveness, whether by the general practitioner, pediatrician, rheumatologist, social worker, psychologist, or psychiatrist.

It is important also to address one's efforts to dealing with the problem, not merely labeling it, i.e., codification of the emotional characteristics of JRA in either the individual child or the group as a whole is less important than efforts to expand the ability of children and parents to cope with the emotions involved with the disease. In this sense, whether emotional events are precipitating factors or results of the disease becomes relatively irrelevant. Social workers, psychologists, and nurses who can assist in liaison with the family's social environment, and physical and occupational therapists who are sensitive to the patient's emotional as well as physical status, may be vital to successful management. It is not clear from existing data whether counselling efforts by these professionals exerts direct long-term benefit, but the information they obtain by close contact can be extremely useful in assisting the primary physician.

The cornerstone of care for the arthritic child and his family is education. Most people regardless of intelligence or education are largely unaware that arthritis exists in childhood, become very anxious when its possibility is discussed, and are totally unfamiliar with the most simple medical and physical therapy approaches. While diagnostic and therapeutic procedures become second nature and appear simple enough to physicians many people have only poorly formed notions about the reasons for what is being required of them.

In our clinic, physicians and social workers spend at least one-half hour in education at the initial consultation visit and then follow this a week later with a "test." The family is forewarned that they will be asked to restate what was said at the first meeting. It appears critical, particularly at the inception of a chronic disease when the physician may be embarking on many years of management, that he be aware of and document how little these educational efforts are accurately perceived or remembered. Repetition of information together with an assessment of how receptive the patient and family are may be very important. One should individualize educational efforts depending upon levels of anxiety and degree of sophistication, i.e., the number of topics presented at a given session may need to be limited so as not to be overwhelming. If in the first month or two of contact the physician can educate and exhibit sensitivity about a wide range of concerns which cause anxiety then he will establish a relationship which will successfully carry through the worst of times for that small percentage of patients who don't respond well physically or psychologically.

The following is a list of common issues which, although simplistic in appearance, are all too frequently ignored, overlooked, or wrongly attributed to some basic fund of knowledge which we presume others to have: (1) What is inflammation, and why is it important to understand it as a fundamental model for arthritis? (2) Why do we use aspirin and why can't it be stopped if the pain goes away? (3) What is the role of pain in causing contractures and why is splinting important? (4) Why are normal as possible activities and periods of rest both important? (5) What kind of school should the child be in? (6) How do you balance the psychologic gains of a regular school setting versus the physical advantages of a "handicapped" school? (7) How do we best educate teachers, friends, relatives, and others to the child's condition and requirements, particularly if the child superficially does not appear disabled? (8) Will disease go away or get worse, and when? (9) What is the outlook for employment opportunities? (10) Will the child become crippled? (11) Will he or she be able to achieve normal sexual relations and have children? (12) Who or what is to blame for the child's developing arthritis? (13) What other medications are available if the child doesn't do well?

It is concerns such as these and the unsatisfying, complex, frequently speculative nature of our responses to such questions that, in our opinion, commonly lead to many of the disordered psychologic reactions which are observed in children with arthritis and in their families. Our inability to answer such critical questions accurately is usually very worrisome to the concerned parent or older child. Answers we can provide to the many questions must be honest and straightforward, including admitting what we don't know. But in stating ignorance or uncertainty, there should remain a sense of physician confidence and competence to deal with any complexities.

Anxiety induced by not knowing what to expect is frequently coupled with fear for the worst, particularly in any large specialty clinic where the most severely disabled are the most obvious, receive a disproportionate share of attention, and have the most frequent appointments. To allay fears of the new patient and parents that the child will become similarly afflicted a detailed discussion of this point is invariably helpful, reduces one common area of anxiety, and helps to alert them all to the physician's sensitivity to issues that they are reluctant to discuss or don't know how to verbalize. It is also important to stress need for the physician and other staff to be good listeners. Frequently patients or their families discharge anxieties by apparently irrelevant, anecdotal chatter. This may be therapeutic as such, but there is commonly a central concern which should be explored more directly.

It is also worthwhile to explain that many well-meaning individuals will offer advice, nostrums, anecdotes about miraculous recoveries, and referrals to clinics which promise fabulous cures. There is often fanfare given to unproven arthritis "cures" in newspapers and magazines, much of which is slanted, prematurely released to the public, or pertains to adult disease forms and is therefore of limited application to children. It is vital that parents and patients be actively encouraged to bring forth and discuss all ideas and suggestions with which they come in contact so that a consistency of information and approach can be achieved.

Fathers of patients deserve special mention. The vast majority of children are brought to our offices by their mothers, and all too frequently the information given by the physician is poorly or inaccurately transmitted to the spouse. Misinformed, dissatisfied, or confused fathers can be a frequent source of sabotage of a physician's best therapeutic efforts. Although occasionally difficult, it is helpful to arrange visits to include the father.

Teenage patients are another group who require special attention and effort. Increased emotional turmoil is expected at this age but psychologic conflicts may be heightened by the presence of arthritis and lead to conscious or unconscious efforts to obstruct a therapeutic program. Medications are often not taken properly, appointments are missed, and exercises not performed because "I really don't have arthritis," "I don't need all this stuff to get better," "I'm in control, I don't need everybody else telling me what to do," or, "what's the use—I'm going to be permanently crippled anway."

It is impossible to overemphasize the importance of a social worker who is committed to in-depth involvement with arthritic patients and their families. Two facts are paramount in our experience: (1) ideally, the social worker should have training and experience in psychologic counselling and a desire to provide this on an individual and group basis, and (2) social workers who divide their efforts among many physicians or several different subspecialty divisions in a teaching hospital are at a disadvantage.

In our setting the social worker is an integral part of the Division of Rheumatology, and attends all teaching and administrative sessions. This greatly assists frequent physician contact for up-dating psychosocial data on specific patients and materially improves the social worker's comprehensive understanding of JRA as a disease process. A psychologist with training and expertise in chronic childhood diseases and a specific commitment to JRA should be an additional member of the team approach.

In this setting ongoing in-depth counselling on an individual patient basis may be crucial to successful management. Additionally, patient and parent group counselling therapy sessions can be extremely helpful, particularly when the participants are allowed to join in common cause against the illness, and where individuals are able to recognize the many common anxieties and questions which they all share. In this situation it is also possible for the psychiatric social worker and/or psychologist to assess therapeutic techniques longitudinally.

Another important therapeutic modality may be in-hospital rehabilitation. The emotional demands which extensive home programs of physical and occupational therapy can place on children and their parents may be exhausting, particularly if, as is frequently so, progress is extremely slow or if the program is successful only in maintaining prior mobility and activities of daily living. In this situation a period of hospitalization in a specialized rehabilitation unit may have numerous advantages. It may provide (1) an emotional respite for the parents from a prolonged period of heavy responsibility, (2) an opportunity for parents and child to communicate concerns independently to interested

264

team members without having to censor their thoughts to conform to the expectations of others involved, (3) a release of tension by shifting physical care responsibilities to professionals and, perhaps most importantly, (4) the opportunity to observe that intensive physical and medical management really can be successful, thus reaffirming faith in the validity of a complex and time-consuming home program.

One could continue endlessly to list important points or observations which exist in, influence, or ameliorate the psychosocial aspects of JRA. Clearly, our perspective and the resources available in a teaching hospital may differ from those of the private practitioner or anyone else who sees only a few children with JRA. However, regardless of the setting detailed education, constant reassessment of what the patient and family truly understand, and awareness of and sensitivity to the emotional consequences of developing JRA, remain vitally important cornerstones in successful management.

REFERENCES

1. Maddison, D., and Raphael, B. Social and psychological consequences of chronic disease in childhood. *Med J Aust.* 2:1265–70, 1971.

2. Brazelton, T.B., Holder, R., and Talbot, B. Emotional aspects of rheumatic fever in children. *J Pediatr.* 43:339–58, 1953.

3. Garrard, S.D., and Richmond, J.B. The psychological aspects of the management of chronic diseases and handicapping conditions in childhood. Edited by H.I. Leif, V.F. Leif, and N.R. Leif. In *Psychological Basis of Medical Practice.* New York: Noeber, 1963, pp. 370–403.

4. Erikson, E.G. *Childhood and Society.* New York: W.W. Norton and Co., Inc., 1950.

5. Mattson, A. Long-term physical illness in childhood: a challenge to psychosocial adaptation. *Pediatrics.* 50:801–11, 1972.

6. Lowit, I.M. Social and psychological consequences of chronic illness in children. *Dev Med Child Neurol.* 15:75–7, 1973.

7. Mattson, A., and Gross, S. Social and behavioral studies on hemophilic children and their families. *J Pediatr.* 68:952–64, 1966.

8. McCollum, A.T., and Gibson, L.E. Family adaptation to the child with cystic fibrosis. *J Pediatr.* 77:571–8, 1970.

9. Green, M. Care of the child with a long-term life threatening illness: some principles of management. *Pediatrics.* 39:441–5, 1967.

10. Cobb, S., Bauer, W., and Whiting, I. Environmental factors in rheumatoid arthritis. *JAMA.* 113:668–70, 1939.

11. King, S.H. Psychosocial factors associated with rheumatoid arthritis. *J Chronic Dis.* 2:287–302, 1955.

12. Wolff, B.B. Current psychosocial concepts in rheumatoid arthritis. *Bull Rheum Dis.* 22:656–61, 1972.

13. King, S.H., and Cobb, S. Psychosocial factors in the epidemiology of rheumatoid arthritis. *J Chronic Dis.* 7:466–75, 1958.

14. King, S.H., and Cobb, S. Psychosocial studies of rheumatoid arthritis: parental factors compared in cases and controls. *Arthritis Rheum.* 2:322–31, 1959.

15. Cobb, S. Contained hostility in rheumatoid arthritis. *Arthritis Rheum.* 2:419–25, 1959.

16. Cobb, S., Schull, W.J., Harburg, E. et al. The intrafamilial transmission of rheumatoid arthritis, I–VIII. *J Chronic Dis.* 22:193–296, 1969.

17. Scotch, N.A., and Geiger, H.K. The epidemiology of rheumatoid arthritis: a review with special attention to social factors. *J Chronic Dis.* 15:1037–67, 1962.

18. Moos, R.H. Personality factors associated with rheumatoid arthritis: a review. *J Chronic Dis.* 17:41–55, 1964.

19. Wolff, B.B. Rheumatoid arthritis: assessment. Edited by J.R. Nichols, and W.H. Bradley. In *Proceedings of a Symposium on the Motivation of the Physically Disabled*. London: National Fund for Research into Crippling Diseases, 1968, pp. 16–20.

20. Cleveland, S.E., and Fisher, S. Comparison of psychological characteristics and physiological reactivity in ulcer and rheumatoid arthritis groups. *Psychosom Med.* 22:283–9, 1960.

21. Moldofsky, H., and Chester, W.J. Pain and mood patterns in patients with rheumatoid arthritis: a prospective study. *Psychosom Med.* 32:309–18, 1970.

22. Wolff, B.B. Factor analysis of human pain responses: pain endurance as a specific pain factor. *J Abnorm Psychol.* 78:292–8, 1971.

23. Meyerowitz, S. The continuing investigation of psychosocial variables in rheumatoid arthritis. Edited by A.G.S. Hill. In *Modern Trends in Rheumatology*. London: Butterworth, 1971.

24. Blom, G.E., and Nicholls, G. Emotional factors in children with rheumatoid arthritis. *Am J Orthopsychiat.* 24:588–601, 1954.

25. Cleveland, S.E., Reitman, E.E., and Brewer, E.J. Psychological factors in juvenile rheumatoid arthritis. *Arthritis Rheum.* 8:1152–8, 1965.

26. Cleveland, S.E., and Brewer, E.J. Psychological aspects of juvenile rheumatoid arthritis. Edited by E.J. Brewer. In *Juvenile Rheumatoid Arthritis*. Philadelphia: W.B. Saunders Co., 1970, pp. 116–31.

27. Meyerowitz, S., Jacox, R.F., and Hess, D.W. Monozygotic twins discordant for rheumatoid arthritis: a genetic, clinical, and psychological study of 8 sets. *Arthritis Rheum.* 11:1–21, 1968.

28. Heisel, J.S. Life changes as etiologic factors in juvenile rheumatoid arthritis. *J Psychosom Res.* 16:411–20, 1972.

29. Grokoest, A.W., Synder, A.I., and Schlaeger, R. *Juvenile Rheumatoid Arthritis*. Boston: Little, Brown and Co., 1962, pp. 31, 101.

30. Rimon, R., Belmaker, R.H., and Ebstein, R.I. Psychosomatic aspects of juvenile rheumatoid arthritis. *Scand J Rheumatol.* 6:1–10, 1977.

31. McAnarney, E.R., Pless, B., Satterwhite, B., and Friedman, S.B. Psychological problems of children with chronic juvenile arthritis. *Pediatrics.* 53:523–8, 1974.

32. Henoch, M.J., Batson, J.W., and Baum, J. Psychosocial factors in juvenile rheumatoid arthritis. *Arthritis Rheum.* 21:229–33, 1978.

INDEX